Fitbit®

by Paul McFedries

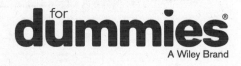
for
dummies®
A Wiley Brand

Fitbit® For Dummies®

Published by: **John Wiley & Sons, Inc.,** 111 River Street, Hoboken, NJ 07030-5774, www.wiley.com

Copyright © 2019 by John Wiley & Sons, Inc., Hoboken, New Jersey

Published simultaneously in Canada

For general information on our other products and services, please contact our Customer Care Department within the U.S. at 877-762-2974, outside the U.S. at 317-572-3993, or fax 317-572-4002. For technical support, please visit https://hub.wiley.com/community/support/dummies.

Wiley publishes in a variety of print and electronic formats and by print-on-demand. Some material included with standard print versions of this book may not be included in e-books or in print-on-demand. If this book refers to media such as a CD or DVD that is not included in the version you purchased, you may download this material at http://booksupport.wiley.com. For more information about Wiley products, visit www.wiley.com.

Library of Congress Control Number: 2019942832

ISBN 978-1-119-59231-0 (pbk); ISBN 978-1-119-59236-5 (ebk); ISBN 978-1-119-59235-8 (ebk)

Manufactured in the United States of America

C10010816_060619

Contents at a Glance

Table of Contents

Introduction

Wait a minute, I hear you thinking, *does the world really need an entire book about Fitbit?* First, whoa, your thinking is loud. Second, yes the world really *does* need a book about Fitbit. Sure, most Fitbit trackers are simple bands that you secure to your favorite wrist and start walking (or running or skipping or whatever). However, that apparent simplicity is only on the surface. Scratch that surface and you uncover an entire world of activity tracking that's much deeper and more powerful than most folks know.

Yes, most Fitbit devices are easy to learn and use, but that up-front ease belies a complex background of features, settings, and customizations that can help you get the most out of your Fitbit. And more sophisticated devices such as the Charge 3 and the Ionic and Versa watches are brimming with buttons and options and apps that come with a learning curve.

Finally, it's one thing to operate your Fitbit, but it's quite another to use your Fitbit to reach a goal. Whether that goal is to get fit, lose weight, eat better, or reduce stress, your Fitbit has settings and features — many of them obscure and hard to find — that can help you get there.

About This Book

So, yep, I wrote a book about Fitbit. Welcome, friend, to *Fitbit For Dummies*, which takes you on a complete tour of the Fitbit ecosystem, from the Fitbit trackers to the Fitbit app to the social features of Fitbit.com. In the end, you'll learn everything you need to know to get the most out of your Fitbit investment — and have a ton of fitness-related fun.

Fitbit For Dummies offers 14 chapters, but just because they appear sequentially, that doesn't mean you have to read them that way. Use the table of contents or index to find the information you need — and dip into and out of the book when you have a question about Fitbit specifically or health and fitness tracking generally.

If your time is limited (or you're just aching to get tonight's TV-watching started), you can also ignore anything marked by the Technical Stuff icon or the information in sidebars (the gray-shaded boxes). Yes, these tidbits are fascinating (if I do say so myself), but they aren't critical to the subject at hand, so you won't miss anything crucial by skipping them.

Within this book, you might see some web addresses breaking across two lines of text. If you're reading this book in print and want to visit one of these web pages, type the web address exactly as it's noted in the text, pretending that any line breaks don't exist. If you're reading this as an e-book, you've got it easy — just tap the web address to be taken directly to the web page.

Foolish Assumptions

This book is for people who are new (or relatively new) to using a Fitbit activity tracker. Therefore, I do *not* assume that you're a Fitbit expert, a Fitbit guru, or a Fitbit whiz. However, I do assume the following:

>> You know how to plug in and connect devices.

>> You have a running Wi-Fi network with an Internet connection.

>> You know the password for your Wi-Fi network.

>> You have an iOS or an Android mobile device (that is, a smartphone or tablet) or a Windows 10 PC.

>> You know how to install and operate apps on your mobile device or PC.

Icons Used in This Book

Like other books in the *Dummies* series, this book's margin has icons, or little pictures, to flag things that don't quite fit into the flow of the chapter discussion. Here are the icons that I use:

REMEMBER

This icon marks text that contains something useful or important enough that you'd do well to store the text somewhere safe in your memory for later recall.

This icon marks text that contains some for-nerds-only technical details or explanations. Feel free to skip this information.

This icon marks shortcuts or easier ways to do things, which I hope will make your life — or, at least, the Fitbit portion of your life — more efficient.

This icon marks text that contains a friendly but unusually insistent reminder to avoid doing something. You have been warned.

Beyond the Book

In addition to what you're reading right now, this product also comes with a free access-anywhere cheat sheet that includes important things you need to know to be healthy and fit, the most useful Fitbit account settings, and a glossary of important health and fitness tracking terms. To get this cheat sheet, go to www.dummies.com/ and type **Fitbit For Dummies Cheat Sheet** in the Search box.

Where to Go from Here

If you've had your Fitbit for a while and you're familiar with the basics, you can probably get away with skipping the first three chapters and diving in to any part of the book that exudes usefulness or interestingness. The chapters present their Fitbit know-how in readily digestible, bite-size tidbits, so feel free to graze your way through the book.

If you and Fitbit haven't met yet — particularly if you're not sure what a Fitbit even *does* — this book has you covered. To get your relationship with Fitbit off to a fine start, I highly recommend reading the book's first three chapters to get some of the basics down cold. From there, you can branch out anywhere you like, safe in the knowledge that you have some survival skills to fall back on!

1

Introducing Fitbit

Discover the benefits and learn the basics of health and fitness tracking.

Check out the available Fitbit devices and learn which one is right for you.

Find out how to configure your Fitbit and install and set up the Fitbit app.

Chapter **1**

Understanding Health and Fitness Tracking

You are a data-generating machine. When you pay with a credit card, drive through an automated toll system, answer an email, or make a call, you leave a steady stream of ones and zeroes in your wake. This so-called *digital exhaust* is the trackable or storable actions, choices, and preferences that you generate as you go about your life. Even when you're just browsing the web, you leave behind not fingerprints but *clickprints* that uniquely identify your surfing behavior and lengthen the paperless trail that documents your electronic self.

All the data you generate is invariably used to make others rich, usually by selling it to advertisers and marketers. Wouldn't it be nice if you could generate data that would help *you*? I'm not talking about data that will make you rich, at least not literally. I'm talking about data that you can use to make yourself healthier, fitter, slimmer, and calmer.

Welcome to the world of health and fitness tracking. In this chapter, I take you on a tour of this world, explore its benefits (and, yes, its few downsides), and introduce you to the types of data you can track. It's all presented from a Fitbit point of view.

Introducing Self-Tracking

From time to time, you might harbor vague worries about oversharing on social networks or being tracked online by ad networks, but you probably don't think about the data shadow you cast wherever you go. However, a growing segment of the population spends a remarkable amount of time and effort trying to generate *more* personal data. While the rest of us are content to step out for a short walk after lunch, these people *count* every step they take. The likes of you and I might groggily estimate the number of hours we slept last night, but these people wear their Fitbits to bed to know exactly how many hours and minutes they slept and what portion of that sleep was spent in the REM (rapid eye movement) state.

I speak of *self-trackers,* people who use technology to acquire, store, and analyze their own life data. Their self-tracking can create detailed records of food, exercise, and location, as well as mood, alertness, overall well-being, and other seemingly non-quantifiable psychological states. This process of self-digitization is almost always enhanced by a Fitbit or similar wearable computing technology that enables the self-monitoring of physiological states and self-sensing of such external data as steps taken and floors climbed. These self-professed data junkies select from a variety of apps and websites that serve as tools for self-quantifying — and that prod them into doing even more of it. It's no wonder, then, that the movement as a whole is often called the *quantified self* and its practitioners are increasingly known as *quantified-selfers* or, simply, *QSers.*

You might think that the point of all this self-scrutiny is just to keep a record of vital stats, but self-trackers are not content with merely tracking a few numbers. Their interest lies in *quantitative assessment:* extracting knowledge from the raw data. They want to put their lives under the *macroscope*, which is the general term for any technology that enhances a person's ability to gather and analyze data. If that data tells you that you're just as bright-eyed and bushy-tailed on days when you managed only five or six hours of sleep, the lesson is clear: You're one of those lucky people who don't need seven or eight hours of sack time. If your heart rate spikes when you sit down to dinner, maybe a little family counseling is in order. In short, by analyzing detailed data over a long time, self-trackers turn themselves into self-experimenters, or perhaps even body hackers. The aim? Nothing more or less than the examined life, albeit one where *examined* means tracked, quantified, recorded, and analyzed.

Why Track Your Health and Fitness?

Self-tracking is a bona fide trend, but is it a bandwagon *you* should jump on? Perhaps you've come to the conclusion that you could be more active, fitter, calmer, and just healthier overall. If so, that's great! But you might also be asking yourself whether you really need to self-track your activities, exercises, food, and sleep. Why go to the trouble? Can't you just do what's necessary and leave it at that?

So many questions! Fortunately, the answers to all of them lead to the simple conclusion that, yes, self-tracking is worth the effort. Why? I've come up with no less than ten reasons:

» Monitoring your progress

» Figuring out what does and doesn't work for you

» Keeping yourself motivated

» Challenging yourself

» Challenging others

» Figuring out what health or fitness activities to try next

» Performing experiments

» Breaking bad habits

» Encouraging good habits

» Learning about yourself

In the next few sections, I fill in the details for each reason.

Putting numbers to feelings: Monitoring your progress

Perhaps the most straightforward reason to track your health and fitness is to measure your progress. Sure, when you first start a new health or fitness regimen, at some point you start to feel better, and in many cases a *lot* better. But that initial massive — and, hence, noticeable — difference soon gives way to smaller — and, hence, not always noticeable — improvements. Before long, it might seem as though you're no longer progressing at all, which is the point at which many people either scale back their lifestyle changes or quit altogether.

The problem here is that determining whether you feel better isn't an exact process, especially when those feelings become subtle. Don't get me wrong: Feeling fitter or healthier is a fantastic reward for all that work you're doing. But for long-term success, you need to back up those subjective feelings with some objective data. To get that objectivity, you need to *measure* your progress by monitoring your activities, exercises, and body composition. That's where your Fitbit comes in, because it gives you a record of what you've done, which you can compare to what you're doing now.

How does that comparison help? Well, if you don't feel all that much better now than you did last month, but your Fitbit tells you that, say, you're averaging two thousand more steps per day or your heart rate is five beats lower, you know you're still heading in the right direction despite how you feel. Oh, and good job, by the way!

Figuring out what does and doesn't work for you

The road to your best self isn't a straight line. Yes, the general direction is clear — move more, eat better, and reduce stress — but the specific route to get there is different for everyone. Ideally, you'll just happen to take the path that's right for you and not head down a bunch of dead-end streets. Ah, but there's the rub: How do you know when you're cruising down the right road and when you're wasting your time on a cul-de-sac? In short (and to finally move on from that now over-done "road" metaphor), how do you know what works for you and what doesn't?

That's where health and fitness tracking shines. After you've used your Fitbit for a while, you end up with a priceless trove of data that you can mine for insights into what has been effective for you in the past. For example, if your main goal is to lose weight, you can analyze your historical data to look for periods when your weight dropped steadily and when your weight stayed the same or even increased. Now you can compare what you were eating, what types of exercise you were doing, how much sleep you were getting, and so on for those different periods. Ideally, you'll start to see patterns in the data that tell you what works and what doesn't.

Keeping yourself motivated

You might think that you don't need to track your health and fitness because all you need to do is set a goal and then work towards it day in and day out, without exception. Well, sure, that would be great if you could manage it, but study after study has shown a hard truth: Willpower doesn't work. By sheer force of will, you can't make yourself do the work necessary to get fit or lose weight or reach whatever you've established as your health or fitness grail.

Does that mean there's no point in even trying? Definitely not! The secret sauce of success here isn't willpower — it's *motivation*. If you're sufficiently motivated to reach your goal, willpower is unnecessary because you'll *want* to do the work you need to do to get where you want to go.

Motivation comes in many forms: an upcoming beach vacation, a future charity run, or a bet with a friend. You can also use your Fitbit to get motivated: If you look back at your historical data and see your daily steps steadily increasing or your weight steadily decreasing, the motivation to keep that trend going is right there.

Not only that, but you can configure your Fitbit with specific daily goals, such as 10,000 steps and 10 floors climbed (see Figure 1-1). Your Fitbit will show your progress towards those goals, motivating you to walk the long way home or take the stairs instead of the elevator to put yourself over the top.

‹ Account	Activity Goals
Daily Activity	
Steps	10,000 steps
Distance	8.05 km
Calories Burned	2,268 cals
Active Minutes	40 minutes
Floors Climbed	10 floors
Hourly Activity Goal	11 hr/day

FIGURE 1-1: Set daily goals for steps, calories burned, floors, and more.

Challenging yourself

One of the main reasons why people fail to reach their health or fitness goals is that they start off well and see some good results, so they just continue what they're doing. That doesn't sound so bad, except that your body has a wonderful way of adapting to most things you throw at it. When you start walking or running or lifting weights, what feels excruciatingly hard at first starts to feel pretty good after you've done it a few times. The exercise is stressing your heart and slightly breaking down your muscles. Once you stop, your body doesn't just repair the damage; it rebuilds your heart and muscles so that they're stronger. That process, which is called *adaptation,* is one of the secrets of getting fit.

Or, I should say, it's one of the secrets of getting fit *if* you slowly and steadily increase the amount of stress you place on your body. If you just keep doing the same old thing, your body will simply adapt to that load and stop improving, which is why all successful health and fitness programs require you to challenge yourself. If you averaged 10 minutes per mile on your runs last week, see if you can run at 9 minutes and 45 seconds per mile this week; if you averaged 10,000 steps a day last month, shoot for 11,000 this month; if you walked 900 miles last year, set your sights on an even 1,000 this year.

How do you know what you did last week, last month, or even last year? Your Fitbit can keep track for you, so it's easy to look back on your historical data and challenge yourself to be a better version of yourself.

Challenging others

Ideally, with the help of your Fitbit, your health and fitness motivation will come from within, but internal motivation isn't all you should look for. *External motivation* — that is, getting other people involved in firing yourself up to exercise or diet or whatever — can be an important part of your new regimen. For example, the simple act of *announcing* your health or fitness goal to friends or family members can do wonders for motivating you to stick to that goal.

How can your Fitbit help here? As I show in Chapter 4, your Fitbit account comes with a ton of social features. For example, after you've connected with some people, the Fitbit app displays a leaderboard that shows who among your friends has done the most steps in the past week, as shown in Figure 1-2. Similarly, Fitbit offers several challenges that you can invite people to participate in. One popular challenge is to see who can take the most steps over the coming weekend.

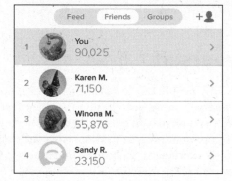

FIGURE 1-2:
See who among your friends has taken the most steps.

Figuring out what comes next

Health and fitness regimens are not — or shouldn't be — static routines. But even if your program includes steady increases and regular challenges (both internal and external), you'll still be faced one day with the "What do I do next?" question. I'm not talking about how many steps you should walk that day or what you should eat. No, this is Big Picture stuff: Adding entirely new types of exercise, cutting out parts of your routine, and so on.

These major changes shouldn't be undertaken willy-nilly. Fortunately, if you've accumulated a decent amount of historical health and fitness data, you can make an informed choice without the willy or the nilly.

For example, if you've been running and cycling, you can examine your previous workouts to see which sport has shown the most improvement. If you feel you've worked equally hard in both but, say, your running performance has improved much faster than your cycling, you might decide to focus more on your running.

Performing experiments

Despite what many so-called gurus will try to sell you, gaining and maintaining health and fitness is not complicated:

WARNING

>> To lose weight, your calories out must exceed your calories in.

>> To eat well, your diet should consist of lots of fresh fruits and vegetables, not too much meat (especially red meat), and little processed food.

>> To get fit, find an activity or sport you like, start easy, and then slowly but steadily increase the duration and intensity.

If you've been sedentary for a long time or have health problems such as heart disease or diabetes, I strongly advise you to see your doctor before beginning any type of exercise program.

>> To sleep well, avoid screen time before bed, go to bed at a regular time, and get at least seven or eight hours of shut-eye.

If you follow these basic guidelines diligently, health and fitness will follow as day follows night. That said, nothing is stopping you from thinking outside this basic health and fitness box. If you run or cycle, for example, you could try adding some workouts on an elliptical machine or a stair-climber to improve leg strength. Or you could add yoga or Pilates sessions to strengthen your core (the muscles around your trunk and pelvis).

However, you need to set up these trials like an experiment. Your Fitbit data will tell you where you are now, and you can then monitor your stats as you add an exercise or activity to see what effect it has.

Breaking bad habits

You form habits by repeatedly making the same choices over time, to the point where you no longer even think about what you're doing. Sit at your desk doing work all day; sit on your couch watching TV all evening; repeat tomorrow and the next day and the day after that. Just like that, you've developed the bad habit of sitting most of the day, and you probably don't even realize it.

Ah, but that's where your Fitbit comes in to save the day. Above all else, a Fitbit is an *activity tracker*, tracking when you move during the day and when you don't.

For example, your Fitbit can track the total number of minutes you're active during the day and the hours during the day when you take at least 250 steps. If your total active minutes is very low and you don't take at least 250 steps most of the hours during the day, you have a bad inactivity habit. But now, thanks to your Fitbit, you *know* you have a bad habit, which is the first step in breaking the habit and getting more active.

Encouraging good habits

Making bad choices over and over, day after day, leads to bad habits, but here's the good news: Making *good* choices over and over, day after day, leads to good habits. Health and fitness tracking can help you get on the good habit path by showing you which activities bring positive results. And seeing those positive results in hard numbers — increased steps, lower heart rate, or a weight closer to your goal — gives you the motivation to keep doing those activities. The result is a virtuous cycle that leads to the formation of good health-and-fitness-enhancing habits.

REMEMBER

Don't expect your good habits to form in a few days or even a few weeks. A 2009 study found that on average is takes people about 66 days to form a habit. So hang in there!

A top-notch tracker will also help you form good habits by giving you small nudges throughout the day. For example, when Fitbit shows you any daily stat, it includes an icon with a partial circle around it, and that circle is completed only when you reach your daily goal. For example, Figure 1-3 shows that today I've taken a bit less than 9,000 steps, and the not-quite-filled-in circle tells me that I'm shy of my goal of 10,000 steps. I want to complete that circle, so I'm motivated to keep moving.

10,000 steps completes this circle

FIGURE 1-3:
The circle associated with each Fitbit stat closes when you've reached your goal.

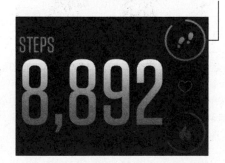

Similarly, most Fitbits will display a notification at ten minutes to the hour if you've yet to meet your hourly goal, which by default is 250 steps, as shown in Figure 1-4. That's just two or three minutes of walking, so why not get out of your seat and move?

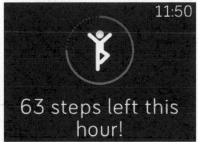

FIGURE 1-4:
Your Fitbit
nudges you if you
haven't taken at
least 250 steps
this hour.

Learning about yourself

A typical health and fitness tracker generates a ton of data. Depending on the device's capabilities, it can track steps, heart rate, floors climbed, distance, pace, active minutes, and calories burned. That wide range of stats has one thing in common: Each piece of data tells you something about yourself. Without a tracker, the days turn into weeks, the weeks turn into months, and the months turn into years, and all the while you almost certainly have only a vague idea of how active you are, how much sleep you're getting, and how well you're eating. And, if you're like most people, even that vague idea is probably an overestimate. Improving your health and fitness means knowing yourself, and the best way to do that is to get some objective data about your activities, workouts, and body composition. That's right in the wheelhouse of any tracker worthy of the name, so if an examined life is your goal, make a health and fitness tracker your tool.

Understanding the Downside of Health and Fitness Tracking

Downside? With all the positive reasons for tracking your health and fitness outlined in the preceding section, could being a self-tracker have any downsides? Yep. Several pitfalls exist, but they are minor and can be easily avoided if you understand them and are mindful of them as you track your activity. Here they are:

>> **Feelings of pressure or stress to meet your daily goals:** Meeting your daily goal for, say, steps taken or active minutes is a great feeling. However, in your

quest to get that feeling, you might end up putting a ton of pressure on yourself. First, remember that although meeting your goals is worthwhile, a relaxed attitude towards those goals is best. Plus, stress can undo many of your health and fitness gains, so there's some twisted irony to self-generating stress *about* those health and fitness gains.

>> **Feelings of guilt, shame, or unworthiness when you don't meet your daily goals:** Your daily activity goals are meant to be a gentle goad that gets you moving and making better choices in your life. These goals are not judgements, however. If you fall short of floors climbed or calories burned, shake it off and resolve to do better tomorrow. Remember that the road to good health and overall fitness is a long one (in fact, it is — or it should be — a life-long one) and doesn't depend on the results of a single day. If you meet your goals most of the time (think of them as "daily-ish" goals), you'll eventually get where you want to go.

>> **Having your daily routines disrupted or controlled by your desire to meet your activity goals:** If by "daily routines" you're talking about prolonged sitting at work or in the evening, being active instead is an upside. However, if an old friend invites you out for a coffee or a meal and you beg off because you need to get in a few thousand more steps to meet your goal, that decision is probably not balanced. Go ahead and meet your friend; you can always reach your goal tomorrow. Better yet, ask your friend to go on a walk with you!

>> **Feeling that an un-tracked activity is a wasted activity:** You go out for a long walk, realize you've forgotten your Fitbit, and no longer enjoy the walk because now the steps and activity time don't "count." Okay, I get it: In an ideal world, you'd never miss a step or a minute or a mile. But in the real world, many activities are untracked. That's fine because it's *way* more important that you are active, even if that activity is now "tracked" only in your head.

>> **Lacking motivation to be active if you don't have your tracker:** This pitfall is related to the preceding one in that an activity undertaken without a tracker isn't real or important because the activity won't generate stats. Without those numbers, you lack the motivation to even do the activity. Remember that your health, not a bunch of stats, is what is real and important. Do the activity anyway because it will get you closer to your long-term goal. Your future healthy and fit self will thank you.

REMEMBER

If you take a walk or perform some other activity without your Fitbit strapped on, your effort doesn't have to go unrecorded. You can always log the activity manually, as described in Chapter 5.

Learning about Health and Fitness Tracking Metrics

A *metric* is a standard that you use to measure something. That standard is usually *quantifiable,* which means that it can be expressed numerically or statistically. Health and fitness tracking — which earlier in this chapter I said was also known as the *quantified-self* movement — is all about metrics and the numbers they generate: steps taken, floors climbed, hours slept, and many more.

Fortunately, these metrics are mostly straightforward, but even apparently simple metrics — such as the number of steps you take in a day — have subtle nuances that you need to understand. I spend the rest of this chapter going through the seven metrics — steps taken, distance covered, floors climbed, active minutes, heart rate, calories burned, and sleep time — tracked by most Fitbits.

REMEMBER

Note I said *most* Fitbits. The simpler Fitbit trackers, such as the Ace for kids and the Zip, only track steps taken, active time, and calories burned. See Chapter 2, to learn more about what metrics each Fitbit device can track.

Steps taken

Fitbit made its name as a simple and easy-to-use step tracker, also known as a *pedometer.* To this day, the number of steps taken daily (see Figure 1-5) remains the device's most iconic and familiar metric. That steps get pride-of-place on your Fitbit isn't surprising because the humble step is an indication of activity. Taking a step means you're not sitting down or standing in one spot, both of which, if done to excess, are bad for your health. You can't get or stay fit without movement, so a step is, well, a step in the right direction.

"Wait a minute," I hear you ask. "If the Fitbit goes on my wrist, how does it know what my feet and legs are doing? Excellent question! The answer is that each Fitbit comes with an *accelerometer,* which is a special sensor designed to detect movement (especially acceleration) and convert that movement into data. A Fitbit can detect steps from your wrist because it assumes that you swing your arms while you move. If a given arm swing's overall motion, speed, acceleration, frequency, and distance surpass a predefined threshold, Fitbit's step-counting algorithm identifies your movement as a step and adds that step to your total.

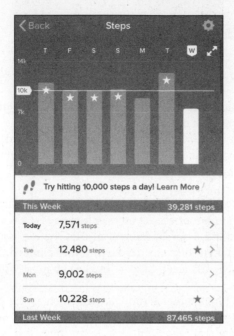

This algorithm works fairly well, particularly because the accelerometer can detect movement along three axes: forward-back, left-right, and up-down. However, you can fool the algorithm in several ways:

>> If your Fitbit-wearing arm is still or moves only a little as you walk (or run), your steps might not get counted. Fortunately, this tendency to miss steps when your arm is still usually doesn't apply when you're pushing a stroller or a shopping cart.

>> In an activity that includes vigorous arm motions without steps — such as shoveling snow and digging holes — those arm motions get counted as steps. I don't view these extra steps as unearned because, let's face it, shoveling and digging are *hard*.

>> If you vigorously swing your arm in a walking or running motion while sitting down or standing in place, those arm swings are counted as steps.

So, yes, it's possible to cheat your step count by swinging your Fitbit-shod arm while not moving. Of course, you would *never* do that because you know as well as I do that you're only cheating yourself, right? *Right?*

Distance covered

Suppose you walk 10,000 steps today and then walk another 10,000 steps six months from now. Suppose, too, that you were exercising regularly during those six months. Does the fact that you did the same number of steps mean that your fitness didn't improve over that time? Not necessarily. If the second time around you covered a greater distance, you got more out of those steps by walking at a faster pace.

Being able to compare how far a given number of steps takes you is, in a nutshell, why the metric of distance covered is important. If you can walk (or run) farther given the same number of steps — or the same elapsed time — your fitness is improving.

Also, distance on its own (that is, without reference to the number of steps involved) is important for runners and cyclists. If you're training for your first 10K race, you need to set up your program to build your distance slowly until you know you can complete the 10K distance.

It might seem weird that a wrist-based device can figure out how far you've traveled during a walk or run (see Figure 1-6). But a Fitbit can calculate distance in not one but three ways:

REMEMBER

>> A Fitbit Ionic watch has an on-board Global Positioning System (GPS) receiver, so it can use that GPS signal to follow your location and calculate your distance automatically.

Both the Ionic and the Versa use GPS only for distance-related activities (such as runs and walks) initiated by the Exercise app (see Chapter 9). The Ionic and the Versa don't use GPS for regularly tracked activities.

>> A Fitbit Versa watch or a Charge 3 or Inspire wristband can connect to your smartphone's GPS receiver and calculate your distance by using that signal.

>> All other Fitbit devices that track distance do so by multiplying the number of steps you take by the length of your stride. Wait, *what!* How can a Fitbit know your stride length? Fitbit calculates stride length automatically by using the height and gender info you supply when you first set up your Fitbit account (see Chapter 3). Actually, Fitbit makes two calculations: your walking stride length and your running stride length.

REMEMBER

If you have your doubts that a stride length calculation based on height and gender can be accurate, not to worry: You can figure out your actual stride lengths and enter them manually, as I explain in Chapter 5.

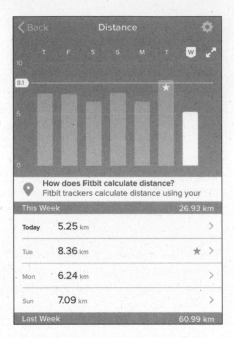

FIGURE 1-6:
Some Fitbits tell you the distance you cover daily.

Floors climbed

Walking along level ground is a fantastic way to get fit and feel better. However, you can quickly and easily kick your fitness program into a higher gear by adding ascents to your walks. These climbs can be the stairs at home or at work, a local street with a steep incline, or a park or similar natural setting with one or more hills. Whatever the ground you're climbing, going up is always harder than staying level, and the steeper the climb the harder the workout.

WARNING

Stairs and hills are tough workouts, even for experienced walkers. If you're just starting your fitness program and you're over 50, or if you suffer from heart disease, kidney disease, diabetes, high blood pressure, or arthritis, talk to your doctor before adding climbs to your workouts.

Certain Fitbit devices can track the number of floors you climb each day (see Figure 1-7). These devices contain a sensor called an *altimeter,* which detects changes in elevation. Whenever the altimeter detects that you've climbed ten feet, it adds a floor to your total. Alas, the altimeter ignores *negative* elevation changes, so you get no credit for going down!

You might be wondering whether you would get climbing credit for cranking up the incline on a treadmill or using a StairMaster? Nope, sorry. The altimeter detects changes in barometric pressure, so your Fitbit has to physically move up in elevation to get credit for a climb.

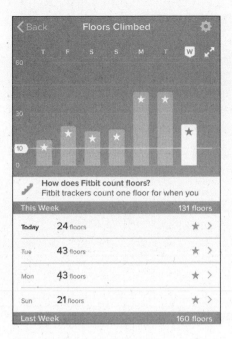

FIGURE 1-7:
A few Fitbits track
the number of
floors you climb
each day.

Active minutes

The worst thing you can do for your health is nothing. Sitting is especially bad, but standing in one place isn't much better. If you want to be fit, the prescription couldn't be simpler: You have to move. Although any movement is good, however, not all types of movement count the same for your long-term health. For example, a leisurely stroll is a fine thing to do, but it's not going to boost your fitness much. Instead, most experts suggest at least 150 minutes of moderate physical activity per week. What does *moderate* mean? Basically, it's any activity that raises your heart rate a little, such as the following:

>> Walking at a brisk pace (at least three miles per hour)

>> Playing tennis

>> Raking leaves and similar yard work

In the Fitbit tracking world, if you perform these types of activities for at least ten minutes, that time is added to your active minutes metric, shown in Figure 1-8. Your Fitbit doesn't know *what* you're doing, of course, but its accelerometer can measure the intensity of your effort, which determines whether the time is counted as active minutes. Even better is a Fitbit with a built-in heart rate monitor (see the next section), because heart rate is a more accurate indicator of an activity's intensity.

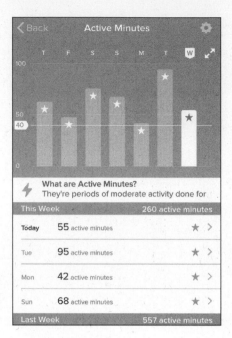

FIGURE 1-8:
Some Fitbits can track your daily number of active minutes.

Heart rate

What's the difference between a languid stroll and a brisk walk, or a slow jog and a fast run? In a word, the stroll and the jog are easier than the walk and the run. Your Fitbit can sense this difference to a certain extent based on the intensity of your arm swings, which tend to be shorter and slower during more leisurely paced activities, and then get longer and faster as you ramp up your speed.

However, another key difference exists between a stroll or jog on one side of the activity spectrum and a brisk walk or run on the opposite end: For the latter, your heart rate — measured in beats per minute (bpm) — climbs higher the faster you go.

Being able to put a number, such as beats per minute, to an effort is more accurate and more trackable over time than arm-swing intensity, which is why some Fitbits come with built-in heart rate monitors.

If you've had any experience with heart rate monitors in the past, you know that the standard setup is a combination of a strap that holds the heart rate sensor to your chest, relatively close to your heart, and a device, such as an exercise watch or smartphone app, that reads the sensor's heart rate data. Using a heart rate monitor is, in short, a hassle.

That hassle disappears when you use a Fitbit to monitor your heart rate, as shown in Figure 1-9, because you don't have to strap on extra devices. Instead, the Fitbit comes with one or more light-emitting diodes (LEDs) on the back (Fitbit calls them PurePulse LEDs). These LEDs reflect onto the skin to detect blood volume changes, which are the telltale signs of your capillaries (small blood vessels) expanding and contracting as your heart beats.

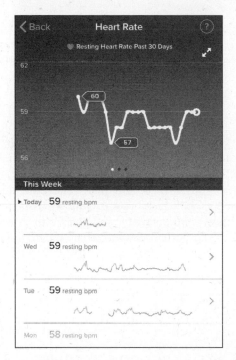

FIGURE 1-9: A few types of Fitbits have onboard heart rate monitors.

Do these LEDs provide an accurate hear rate? For the most part, yes, particularly when you're at rest or moving moderately. Heart rate detection problems can crop up during higher-intensity exercise and during activities that require frequent wrist bending (such as weight lifting) or vigorous, non-rhythmic arm movements (such as martial arts). I talk more about heart rate monitoring in Chapter 7.

Calories burned

If your interest in self-tracking is mostly as an aid to losing weight or maintaining your current weight, tracking the calories you burn each day is crucial. The direction your weight goes depends mostly on calories:

>> **To lose weight:** The calories you take in during the day must be less than the calories you burn.

>> **To maintain weight:** The calories you consume must be roughly the same as the calories you burn.

Some confounding factors exist; for example, muscle weighs more than fat, so any activity that replaces fat with muscle will often cause you to gain weight. But in general, the difference between calories in and calories out determines whether and how your weight changes.

Fitbit enables you to monitor the "calories in" part of the equation by its daily food log, where you enter what you consume by hand or by scanning a food item's barcode, if it has one. From this information, Fitbit automatically calculates the total calories from its food database. For more details about tracking food, see Chapter 10.

For the "calories out" part of the calculation, Fitbit first determines the rate at which you burn calories to perform standard bodily functions such as your heart-beat, breathing, and brain activity. This calculation is called you basal metabolic rate (BMR), and Fitbit determines it based on your height, weight, age, and gender. Fitbit also estimates calories burned based on the intensity and duration of activities and exercises, as well as your heart rate, if your Fitbit measures that. With these three measurements — BMR, activity, and heart rate (if available) — your Fitbit tracks your daily calories burned as a metric, as shown in Figure 1-10.

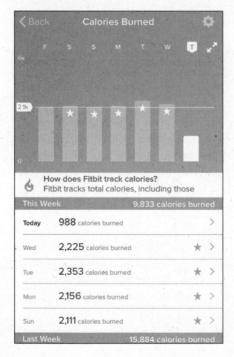

FIGURE 1-10:
Most Fitbits use your BMR and activities to track daily calories burned.

Sleep time

If you don't get enough sleep on a particular night, you'll probably still be able to function normally the next day, perhaps with a few extra yawns. But if you don't get enough sleep for many nights in a row, numerous studies have shown that you'll experience some significant physical and cognitive decline.

Suppose that you try to counteract the nastiness of chronic sleep deficit by going to bed at 11 p.m. and waking up at 7 a.m. Eight hours of solid sack time means problem solved, right? Not so fast. Sure, you might have been *in bed* for eight hours, but were you sleeping the entire time? Or were you restless during the night? Did you rouse yourself one or more times? Did you wake up at 6:30 a.m. and lie there until your alarm went off at 7:00 a.m.? You may have actually slept as little as six or seven hours. Problem most definitely not solved.

Knowing how much sleep you're really getting is difficult because being objective about the quality of your sleep is difficult. Fortunately, your Fitbit is here to help by monitoring your sleep and reporting the results as the amount of time you were awake, restless, and asleep, as shown in Figure 1-11. Even better, if your Fitbit has a heart rate monitor, it can break down your sleep time into sleep stages, such as light sleep or REM sleep. I explain how the Fitbit tracks sleep patterns in Chapter 6.

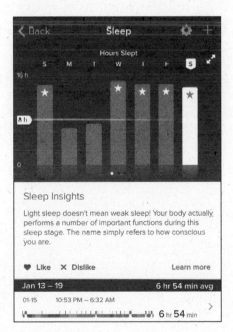

FIGURE 1-11:
Most Fitbits can track your daily sleep time.

Chapter **2**

Choosing a Fitbit

t's certainly possible to track certain aspects of your life by hand. Stats such as activities performed, time spent exercising, heart rate, weight, and foods you eat are all eminently hand-trackable for the dedicated. But lots of metrics are much harder — perhaps even impossible — to track on your own: steps taken, calories burned, and distance covered, to name a few. All of these more difficult stats are a breeze for a device dedicated to tracking your health and fitness, such as a typical Fitbit.

If you're sold on the idea of self-tracking but don't want to do it manually and don't yet have a device to do the tracking, you've come to the right place. In this chapter you explore the world of Fitbit tracking devices, from simple bands that you slap on your wrist and more or less forget about to sophisticated watches that can nearly run your life. You learn about the different device types, see descriptions of each current Fitbit device, compare features, and then figure out which one to get.

Understanding the Different Fitbit Types

When you hear the word "Fitbit," you might conjure up an image of a simple band that goes around a person's wrist and magically gives that person license to tell everyone within earshot how many steps he's taken that day. That's an accurate image, as far as it goes, but Fitbit devices have come a long way since the release in 2009 of the original tracker, which was called, appropriately enough, Tracker. Now Fitbit divides its main activity tracking products into three categories: clip-ons, wristbands, and watches. In the next three sections I take you through the distinguishing features in each category.

Clip-On

A *clip-on activity tracker* comes with a metal or plastic clip that uses tension to hold the tracker in place when the device is attached to a belt, a pocket, or another item of clothing. Figure 2-1 shows an example that offers a small screen displaying the tracker's activity data, which is usually just steps and calories, plus a clock.

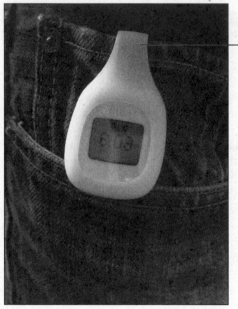

This part clips on a belt or a pocket

FIGURE 2-1:
An example of a clip-on activity tracker.

Photo by Steven Walling via Wikipedia, licensed under CC BY-SA 3.0

Fitbit started off making only clip-ons back in 2009 with the original Fitbit Tracker. These days, the company offers a single clip-on tracker called the Fitbit Zip (shown in Figure 2-1), which I talk about in more detail later in the chapter.

Although almost all clip-on trackers come with a screen that shows activity such as the number of steps taken so far today, checking the screen is often inconvenient, so most people check this type of tracker infrequently. That inconvenience is the main reason why the activity tracking world has moved on to the other two tracker types: the wristband and the watch.

Wristband

A *wristband activity tracker* is worn around either the left or right wrist. Most such trackers come with two components:

» The tracker device, which might or might not include a screen

» A wristband to which the tracker attaches

REMEMBER

Some trackers — notably Fitbit's Flex 2 device — can detach from the wristband and connect with accessories that enable the tracker to be worn as a pendant or a bangle. Fitbit doesn't make such accessories, but many third parties offer them.

Figure 2-2 shows Fitbit's original wristband-type tracker, the Fitbit Flex, which the company released in 2013.

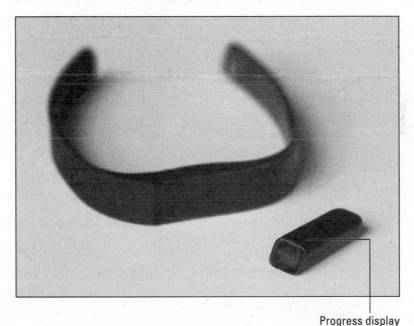

FIGURE 2-2:
The original Fitbit Flex wristband.

Progress display

Photo by MorePix via Wikipedia, licensed under CC BY-SA 3.0

The major advantage of a wristband tracker versus a clip-on is that it's easier to monitor the display to track your progress. The Flex doesn't have a screen (nor does its modern replacement, the Flex 2, which I talk about later in this chapter). Instead, a series of light-emitting diodes (LEDs) illuminate as you progress towards your daily step goal (which is why Fitbit calls these lights the *progress display*). One light means you've reached 25 percent of your goal, two lights indicates 50 percent, and so on.

These days, most people choose a wristband tracker with a screen that enables the wearer to see the current time or daily activity stats, such as steps taken or calories expended. Modern Fitbit wristband models such as the Ace, Charge 3, Inspire, and Inspire HR all come with displays.

Watch

A *watch activity tracker* looks and works much like a regular watch, but it can also do the following:

>> Display many different activity metrics, including steps, calories, distance, sleep data, and heart rate

>> Access the global positioning system (GPS), either directly or by using the GPS signals from a connected smartphone or similar device

>> Run apps that perform special tasks, such as recording a run or swim workout

>> Access third-party content and services, such as music, podcasts, online training sites, and voice-activated assistants such as Amazon's Alexa

This impressively wide range of features is why this type of device is often called a *smart watch* (or smartwatch) or a *super watch*.

Figure 2-3 shows Fitbit's original watch-style activity tracker, the Fitbit Surge, which the company released in 2014. That model has been superseded by the Ionic, and Fitbit also offers a slightly lower-end watch called the Versa (both of which I talk about in the next section).

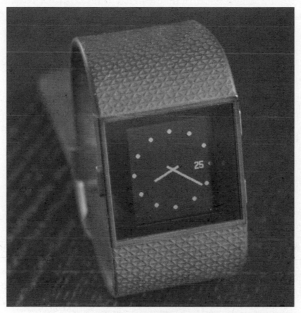

Reviewing Fitbit Trackers

Fitbit offers a surprisingly large collection of activity tracking devices, including simple clip-on trackers, full-featured watches, and even a scale. To give you a sense of the entire lineup, the next few sections offer short summaries of what each Fitbit can do.

Ace

The Ace (and the updated Ace 2, which was announced but not yet released when this book went to press) is a wristband-style tracker (see Figure 2-4) designed for kids aged eight years old and up. The Ace tracks a few useful health and fitness metrics, including steps, active minutes, and sleep duration, and it enables kids to track their progress, challenge their friends, set activity goals, and win rewards and badges for achieving those goals.

What sets the Ace apart from the other Fitbit offerings is its kid-centric focus, which includes a collection of fun clock faces, child-size wristbands (it comes with two: one larger and one smaller), and a Kid View for the Fitbit app, which presents a scaled-down version of standard app features (as well as a Parent View that enables parents to monitor their children's activity and ensures that only parents control each child's Fitbit account).

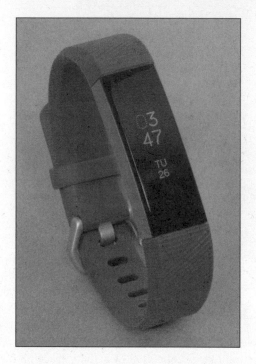

FIGURE 2-4:
The Fitbit Ace wristband tracker.

WARNING

Although Fitbit describes the Ace as "showerproof," it is *not* waterproof. It is, instead, merely *water-resistant*, meaning that it should survive most spills and splashes, sweaty workouts, and even short exposures to light rain (that's what the *shower* in *showerproof* is referring to), but it's not meant to be used when swimming, bathing, or lingering under a hot shower.

Aria 2

The Aria 2 is a departure for Fitbit because it isn't something you wear. Instead, it's a weighing scale — Fitbit calls it a *smart scale* — that you step on (see Figure 2-5).

The Aria 2 shows not only your weight (in pounds, kilograms, or stone) but also your body fat percentage and your body mass index. (If these terms are mere gobbledygook to you, not to worry: I explain all in Chapter 8.) The Aria 2 supports up to eight different users and uses Wi-Fi to sync your weigh-ins with your Fitbit account, which enables you to monitor the effect your activity has on your weight and body fat.

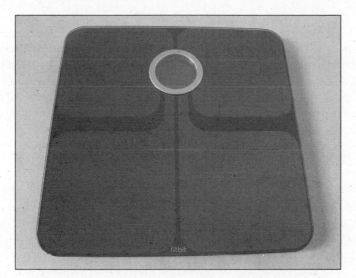

FIGURE 2-5:
The Fitbit Aria 2
weighing scale.

Charge 3

The Charge 3 is a wristband tracker (see Figure 2-6) crammed with features for enhancing not only your health and fitness tracking but the rest of your life as well. The just-the-right-size display shows the time and the usual tracking suspects, including steps, distance, floors climbed, calories burned, sleep, and total active minutes. The Charge 3 has a built-in wrist-based heart rate monitor, so you also see your real-time heart rate and get heart-rate-related features such as heart rate zones, cardio fitness level, and sleep stages.

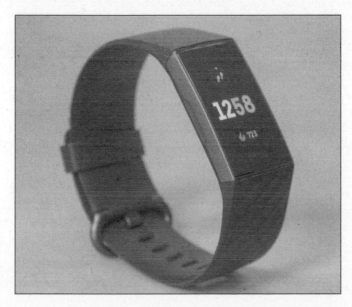

FIGURE 2-6:
The Fitbit Charge
3 wristband
tracker.

The Charge 3 tracker also supports SmartTrack for automatic exercise recognition and can track real-time pace and distance by connecting to the GPS on your smartphone. The Charge 3 comes with several apps that enable you to set more than a dozen exercise modes, perform guided breathing sessions, and set alarms, countdown timers, and use a stopwatch. The device is waterproof to 50 meters, so you can use it to track your swims and leave it on while you take a shower.

Flex 2

The Flex 2 is the successor to Fitbit's original Flex wristband-type tracker and is the simplest — and the least expensive — of the Fitbit devices. Like the Flex, the Flex 2 doesn't have a screen. Instead, it offers a progress display consisting of five LED lights that illuminate as you get closer to your daily step goal. When you reach your goal, one of the lights flashes green to celebrate.

That same LED flashes blue when you receive a call or text notification, magenta when you get a reminder to move, and red when the device's battery is low. The Flex 2 supports sleep tracking, SmartTrack, and silent alarms. If you're a swimmer, you'll be glad to hear that the device is waterproof down to 50 meters.

Inspire

If you want a slim, wristband-style tracker with a screen, the Inspire is worth checking out (as well as its close cousin, the Inspire HR, described in the next section). With a thin wristband and an equally thin display (identical to the one shown in Figure 2-7), the Inspire doesn't take up much wrist room, but its tappable screen offers the date and time; activity stats such as steps, calories burned, active minutes, distance, and hourly activity (that is, taking at least 250 steps each hour); and health metrics such as time asleep, water consumption, and weight.

The Inspire also supports Fitbit's SmartTrack feature, which automatically recognizes certain activities, such as walks and runs of at least 15 minutes, and adds them to your exercise list for the day. The Inspire also has silent alarms, a countdown timer, and a stopwatch, and can display smartphone notifications.

Inspire HR

The Inspire HR, shown in Figure 2-7, is a wristband-type activity tracker that looks similar to the Inspire. The main difference between the Inspire and the Inspire HR is that the latter comes with a built-in heart rate monitor that shows your ticker's beats per minute in real time. The Inspire HR monitors your heart rate at the wrist, so no bulky and inconvenient chest strap is required. Nice.

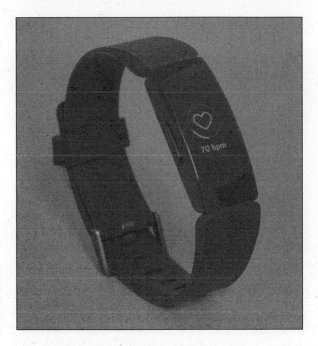

FIGURE 2-7:
The Fitbit
Inspire HR
wristband
tracker.

The Inspire HR also includes a number of features that you won't find in the Inspire, including sleep stages, swim tracking, exercise modes, cardio fitness level tracking, and support for using the GPS on a connected smartphone.

That heart rate data also gives the Inspire HR three other features that aren't in the Inspire:

>> **Heart rate zones:** Heart rate ranges that you can target during exercise. I talk about the importance of heart rate zones in Chapter 7.

>> **Cardio fitness level:** A cardio fitness score that you can track over time to see how your cardiovascular fitness is improving. For the details, see Chapter 9.

>> **Sleep stages:** The amount of time you spend each night in light, deep, and rapid eye movement (REM) sleep. For more about these different types of sleep, check out Chapter 6.

Ionic

The Ionic is a watch-style tracker (see Figure 2-8) and Fitbit's flagship device. This baby is loaded with just about every feature offered by Fitbit: clock, activity tracking, sleep tracking, SmartTrack, exercise modes, and smartphone notifications.

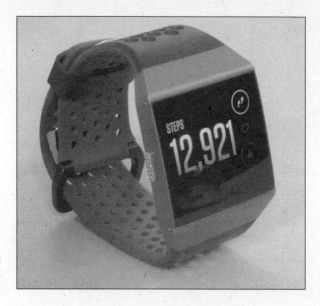

FIGURE 2-8:
The Fitbit Ionic
watch tracker.

The Ionic has a built-in heart rate monitor and Global Positioning System (GPS) receiver, a large and sharp display, a five-day battery life, and storage for more than 300 songs. In addition, it's waterproof to 50 meters. The Ionic comes with a number of apps for guided breathing, alarms and timers, the weather, and personalized coaching, but it also supports all third-party Fitbit apps. It's the most expensive of the Fitbit devices, but there's not much that the Ionic can't do.

Versa

Similar to the Ionic, the Versa is a watch-type tracker. However, the Versa lacks a built-in GPS (you can still get real-time pace and distance by connecting the Versa to a smartphone), has a shorter battery life of four days, and is (at least in my opinion) less stylish. However, the Versa *does* support a long list of features and is $70 cheaper than the Ionic.

Fitbit also offers the Versa Lite Edition, which is a scaled-down version of the regular Versa that's $40 cheaper but doesn't tracks floors climbed or swims, doesn't offer onscreen workouts, and doesn't support Fitbit Pay.

Zip

The Zip, which was shown previously in Figure 2-1, is Fitbit's only clip-on tracker and its simplest device. The teensy display shows only the time, plus your steps, activity minutes, and calories burned. Yep, that's the end of the list of features!

The biggest plus that the Zip has going for it is battery life, which Fitbit says can be as long as six months. If you want a set-it-and-forget-it tracker, the Zip might be for you.

Deciding on a Fitbit Tracker

If you still haven't decided on a Fitbit as a treat for yourself or to get as a gift for a friend or family member, I can't say that I blame you: You have so many choices! Not to worry because I'm here to help. In the rest of this chapter, I go through some useful questions to ask yourself and present a more detailed look at the features that come with each Fitbit activity trackers.

Figuring out what you require in a tracker

You no doubt want an activity tracker to, well, track your activities: steps taken, distance travelled, calories burned, floors climbed, and minutes active. Almost all Fitbit trackers except the Aria 2 have you covered (with a few exceptions; see Table 2-1, a bit later in this chapter). So to decide on a tracker, you need to go beyond basic activity-tracking and ask yourself a few questions:

>> **Are you on a budget?** I get it: $270 (the suggested price of an Ionic watch) is a lot of money for an activity tracker. (All prices quoted here are for the United States and were current as of Spring 2019 when this book went to press.) If you want (or need) to spend two figures instead of three, the Inspire wristband tracker at $69.95 is your cheapest bet.

>> **Do you need to monitor your heart rate?** When you get a built-in heart rate monitor, you can not only see your resting heart rate in real-time but also track your heart rate during exercise. You also get Fitbit features such as heart rate zone, cardio fitness level, and sleep stages. If that all sounds good to you, the Inspire HR might be the way to go. However, if you don't mind spending an extra $50, I suggest the Charge 3, which offers a bigger screen and a few more features than the Inspire HR (which might be why the Charge 3 is Fitbit's bestselling tracker). Note, too, that the Ionic and Versa watches also come with a built-in heart rate monitor.

>> **Will the tracker be used by a kid?** Children can certainly use simpler trackers such as the Inspire and the Zip, but it's worth giving the Ace a good look because it was designed by Fitbit with kids in mind.

>> **Do you want to track non-cardio workouts such as weight sessions and yoga classes?** The SmartTrack feature on many Fitbit devices will automatically recognize certain exercises that last at least 15 minutes, such as walks, runs, bike rides, and swims. However, other fitness routines such as martial arts sessions, weight workouts, and yoga or similar movement classes might not be recognized. To ensure that fitness activities that aren't automatically recognized get tracked, use the Exercise app to tell Fitbit the exercise you're currently doing. This app is available with the Charge 3, Inspire HR, Ionic, and Versa devices.

>> **Do you want to track real-time pace and distance without having to carry your smartphone with you?** When you're running or cycling, the two most important metrics (besides your overall time, of course) are your current pace — usually measured in minutes per mile or kilometer — and the distance you cover during the workout. Most Fitbit devices can measure distance based on your estimated stride length. But for more accurate distance measures and to calculate your real-time pace, you need access to GPS, and Fitbit devices such as the Charge 3, Inspire HR, and the Versa do the GPS thing by connecting to a nearby smartphone's GPS signal. If you'd prefer to carry just your Fitbit on your run or ride, that Fitbit needs to be an Ionic watch, which has a GPS receiver built-in.

>> **Do you want to track your swims?** All Fitbit trackers are at least water-resistant, which means they won't go kaput if they get splashed or if you get caught in a light rain. If you want to use your Fitbit for swimming, however, you need a tracker that's fully waterproof. Fitbit offers five waterproof devices that support swim tracking: Charge 3, Flex 2, Inspire HR, Ionic, and Versa.

>> **Do you want a long battery life?** All Fitbit trackers run on a battery charge, and the number of days that charge lasts depends on how you use your device. For the majority of people, most Fitbit trackers can go for about four or five days without needing recharging. If you want longer battery life than that, you need to look at either the Inspire or the Inspire HR, which can go about five days between charges, or the Zip clip-on tracker, which can last up six months without needing to be plugged in.

>> **Do you need access to music, podcasts, and other third-party content?** Most people want an activity tracker that does nothing but track their activities. But if you're thinking that a device that will be strapped onto your wrist all day should also do other things, such as play music or podcasts (using a connected speaker) and offer games and other third-party content, you need to get a Fitbit watch — either the Ionic or the Versa will do.

Comparing Fitbit activity tracker features

I provided a basic description of the features of each Fitbit tracker earlier in this chapter (see "Reviewing Fitbit Trackers"). However, when deciding which tracker to get, it helps to see a side-by-side comparison of all the possible features. Sounds like a lot of work, right? Well, it is — but you're worth it. Table 2-1 presents just such a comparison for every device from the Ace through the Zip (although it doesn't include the Aria 2 smart scale, because it's not an activity tracker).

TABLE 2-1   ## Fitbit Feature Comparison

Feature	Ace	Inspire HR*	Charge 3	Flex 2	Ionic	Versa	Zip
Price**	$99.95	$99.95°	$149.95	$59.95	$269.95	$199.95	$69.95
Type	Wristband	Wristband	Wristband	Wristband	Watch	Watch	Clip-on
Activity Features							
Step tracking	Yes	Yes	Yes	Yes	Yes	Yes	Yes
Activity tracking	Yes	Yes	Yes	Yes	Yes	Yes	Yes
Hourly activity	Yes	Yes	Yes	Yes	Yes	Yes	–
Calories burned	–	Yes	Yes	Yes	Yes	Yes	Yes
Floors climbed	–	Yes*	Yes		Yes	Yes	
Reminders to move	Yes	Yes	Yes	Yes	Yes	Yes	–
Exercise Features							
SmartTrack (auto exercise recognition)	–	Yes	Yes	Yes	Yes	Yes	–
Exercise modes	–	Yes*	Yes	–	Yes	Yes	–
On-screen workouts	–	–	–	–	Yes	Yes	–
Pace and distance with built-in GPS	–	–	–	–	Yes	–	–
Pace and distance with phone GPS	–	Yes*	Yes	–	–	Yes	–
Swim tracking	–	Yes*	Yes	Yes	Yes	Yes	–

(continued)

TABLE 2-1 *(continued)*

Feature	Ace	Inspire HR*	Charge 3	Flex 2	Ionic	Versa	Zip
Cardio fitness level	–	Yes*	Yes	–	Yes	Yes	–
Health Features							
Heart rate tracking	–	Yes*	Yes	–	Yes	Yes	–
Sleep tracking	–	Yes	Yes	Yes	Yes	Yes	–
Sleep stages	–	Yes*	Yes	–	Yes	Yes	–
Female health tracking	–	Yes	Yes	–	Yes	Yes	–
Guided breathing sessions	–	Yes*	Yes	–	Yes	Yes	–
Other Features							
Clock	Yes	Yes	Yes	–	Yes	Yes	Yes
Alarms	–	Yes	Yes	Yes	Yes	Yes	–
Stopwatch	–	Yes	Yes	–	Yes	Yes	–
Countdown timer	–	Yes	Yes	–	Yes	Yes	–
Call notifications	–	Yes	Yes	Yes	Yes	Yes	–
Text notifications	–	Yes	Yes	Yes	Yes	Yes	–
Smartphone app notifications	–	Yes	Yes	Yes	Yes	Yes	–
Quick replies	–	–	Yes	–	Yes	Yes	–
Calendar alerts	–	Yes	Yes	–	Yes	Yes	–
Fitbit apps	–	–	–	–	Yes	Yes	–
Music storage	–	–	–	–	Yes	Yes	–
Fitbit Pay	–	–	Yes	–	Yes	Yes	–
Waterproof	–	Yes	Yes	Yes	Yes	Yes	–
Battery life (days)	*5*	*5*	*7*	*5*	*5*	*4*	*180*

* Features marked with an asterisk (*) are available only on the Inspire HR, not the Inspire.

** Prices are in US dollars and were current when this book went to press in the spring of 2019.

° The suggested retail price of the Inspire is $69.95.

IN THIS CHAPTER

» Taking the first steps with your new Fitbit device

» Treating yourself to a Fitbit account

» Getting familiar with the Fitbit app

» Setting up the Fitbit app to suit your style and goals

» Learning some useful techniques for working with your Fitbit

Chapter **3**

Getting Started

Well begun is half done, as the old saying goes, so it pays to set aside some time at the start of your soon-to-be illustrious Fitbit career to learn some crucial basics and take care of important details. Sure, the all-but-impossible-to-resist temptation is to rip your shiny, new Fitbit out of its packaging, slap it on your wrist, and start stepping out. I did exactly that when I got my first Fitbit, and as fun as it was to jump into the deep end of the self-tracking world, I soon found myself perplexedly scratching my head over a few things.

This chapter helps you avoid the same sorry fate by showing you some basics, such as charging your device, setting up a Fitbit account, and installing the Fitbit app and connecting it to your device. You also learn some useful account and app customizations, set up your health and fitness goals, and find out how to work with your device. It might seem like a lot of effort compared to just putting on your tracker, but you'll thank me in the end.

Charging Your Fitbit

Right out of the box, your Fitbit's battery is partially charged, so your first order of business is to get your device's battery topped up and ready for action. How you charge your Fitbit depends on the device:

» **Ace, Alta, Alta HR, Charge 3:** Plug the USB end of the charging cable into a powered USB slot. Clip the other end of the cable to the back of your Fitbit, making sure that the pins inside the clip align with the gold connectors on the back of the Fitbit. When the charging cable is connected properly, the device vibrates briefly and the Fitbit logo or the battery icon appears.

» **Aria 2:** The Aria ships with three AA batteries preinstalled, so no charging is required. To enable the initial power-up of the Aria, pull to remove the plastic tab poking out of the battery compartment.

» **Flex 2:** Plug the USB end of the charging cable into a powered USB slot. Remove the Flex 2 from its wristband, clip the other end of the charging cable to the back of your Fitbit, making sure that the pins inside the clip align with the gold connectors on the back of the Fitbit. When the charging cable is connected properly, the device vibrates briefly and the charge indicator lights blink.

» **Inspire, Inspire HR, or Ionic:** Plug the USB end of the charging cable into a powered USB slot. Hold the other end of the cable near the back of the tracker and let the built-in magnet guide the cable's connector into the tracker's port. When the tracker is connected properly, the Fitbit logo and then the current battery percentage appear onscreen.

» **Versa:** Plug the USB end of the charging cable into a powered USB slot. Pinch the spring clip on the other end of the cable and then lay the Versa into the charging cradle with the front of the watch facing you and the gold contacts on the back of the watch aligned with the pins in the cradle. Release the spring clip. When the Versa is connected properly, you see the current battery percentage onscreen.

» **Zip:** The Zip comes with a CR2025 battery that you need to install, so no charging is required. To install the battery, insert the battery door tool into the slot on the back of the Zip, rotate counterclockwise until the arrow on the door aligns with the unlock icon on the device, and then remove the battery door. Insert the battery, making sure the side with the + icon is facing you. Align the arrow on the battery door with the unlock icon on the back of the Zip, and then use the battery door tool to rotate the door clockwise until the door arrow aligns with the lock icon.

REMEMBER

For Fitbit devices that require charging, allow two or three hours for the charge to complete before using the device.

Getting the Fitbit App

Here are a few questions about Fitbit that may or may not have occurred to you:

>> Fitbits such as the Ace and the Alta display only your daily stats. How can you configure these devices?

>> Your Fitbit seems happy to track your health and fitness numbers, but is there a way to save each day's results?

>> You gave Fitbit some vital statistics (such as your weight) during the setup process, but how do you change that info later?

>> Fitbit can play music, but how does Fitbit know whether to use your own music or a service such as Deezer or Pandora?

These are great questions, and they all have the same answer: Use the Fitbit app, which is a program that you download to your smartphone, tablet, or PC. The Fitbit app connects to your Fitbit device, which then enables you to configure the device, save your stats, change your personal info, and set up third-party services such as a music provider.

Okay, so what do you need to get the Fitbit app? Either of the following:

>> **A smartphone or tablet that meets one of these qualifications:**

• An Android phone or tablet running Android 5 or later

• An iPhone or iPad running iOS 10 or later

• A Windows 10 PC running Windows 10 version 1607 or later

>> If you have one of these devices, go to your device's app store, search for the Fitbit app, and install it.

>> **An older Windows PC or a Mac:** If you don't have a device that can run the Fitbit app, you can still do the Fitbit thing using an application called Fitbit Connect, which works with a variety of operating systems, including the following:

• All versions of macOS

• OS X Leopard or later

- Windows XP

- Windows 7

- Windows 8.1

- Early versions of Windows 10 (that is, versions prior to 1607).

» Point your web browser to www.fitbit.com/setup, click the Download link, and then double-click the downloaded file to install Fitbit Connect on your computer.

Either way, your first app task is to sign up for a Fitbit account, as I describe next.

Signing Up for a Fitbit Account

When you first open the Fitbit app (or Fitbit Connect), you're prompted to sign up for a Fitbit account (or to log in with your Fitbit credentials, if you already have an account). Figure 3-1 shows the initial screen that appears for the Fitbit app on an iPhone.

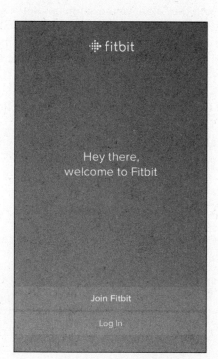

FIGURE 3-1: The iPhone version of the Fitbit app's initial screen.

Follow these steps to join Fitbit:

1. **Select Join Fitbit.**

   If you already have a Fitbit account, select Log In instead, enter your account email and password, and then select Log In again. You're done here, so feel free to merrily skip over the rest of these steps.

   The app displays a list of Fitbit devices.

2. **Select the type of Fitbit device you're setting up.**

   In some cases, you see a second screen that displays a list of device subtypes. If you see such a screen, select the subtype of the device you're setting up.

3. **Select a button to continue:**

   • *Android:* Select Set Up Your Fitbit *Device*, where *Device* is the name of the device you selected in Step 2. The Fitbit app displays the Let's Get Started screen, which is similar to the screen shown in Figure 3-2 except that it doesn't include the First Name and Last Name fields.

   • *iOS:* Select Set Up. The Fitbit app displays the Enter Your Account Details screen, as shown in Figure 3-2.

   • *Windows 10:* Select Set Up Your *Device*, where *Device* is the name of the device you selected in Step 2. The Let's Get Started screen appears, which is similar to the screen shown in Figure 3-2, without the First Name and Last Name fields.

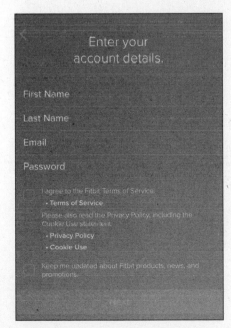

FIGURE 3-2:
The Enter Your Account Details screen as it appears on an iPhone.

4. **Enter the email address and password you want to use for your Fitbit account.**

If you're running the Fitbit app on an iOS device, enter your first and last names, as well.

5. **Select the I Agree to the Fitbit Terms of Service check box.**

6. **(Optional) If you want to receive the latest Fitbit announcements and special offers, select the Keep Me Updated about Fitbit Products, News and Promotions check box.**

7. **Select Next.**

If you're using the Windows 10 version of the Fitbit app, select Create Account, instead.

If you're using the iOS version of the app, on the next screen tap Let's Go.

The Fitbit app prompts you to enter some info about yourself, such as your birthday, height, weight, and sex. How you enter this data depends on the version of the app. In the iOS version, you run through a series of screens. In the Android and Windows 10 version, you see the About You screen. Figure 3-3 shows the About You screen that appears in the Windows 10 version of the Fitbit app.

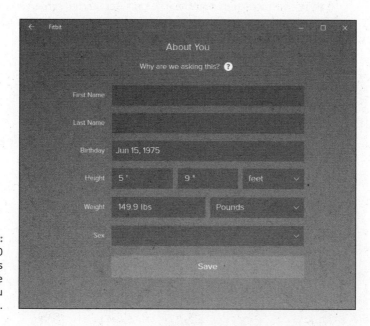

FIGURE 3-3: Windows 10 users see this version of the About You screen.

Why does Fitbit want to know such intimate details about your life? It's all in the service of enabling you to better track your health and fitness. Knowing your age, height, weight, and sex means Fitbit can generate more accurate statistics such as how far you walk or run each day and the number calories you burn during this activity. You might be tempted to fudge the data a bit, but you'll get more out of your Fitbit investment if you enter accurate data.

8. **Enter your personal data, then select Create Account (iOS), Create an Account (Android), or Save (Windows 10).**

   If you see an alert asking you to turn on Bluetooth, go ahead and select OK.

   The app displays the Fitbit terms and policies.

9. **Pretend to read the legalese and then tap I Agree.**

   The Fitbit app now starts the process of configuring the device you selected way back in Step 2. I talk about this configuration stage in more detail in the section that follows.

Connecting Your Fitbit Device

The setup process has two main stages: getting you signed up for a Fitbit account and configuring your Fitbit device. I went through the steps for getting your Fitbit account in the preceding section, so now it's time to look at configuring your device.

If you're setting up a Fitbit Ace for a child, you don't set up the device directly as I describe in this section. Instead, you need to create a family account and then add your child's Ace from there. See Chapter 4 for details.

First, you need to check the following:

>> Make sure your Fitbit device is charging, as I described earlier in the "Charging Your Fitbit" section.

>> For most Fitbit devices, make sure the device that's running the Fitbit app has Bluetooth enabled.

>> For some Fitbit devices — particularly the Ionic and Versa watches and the Aria 2 smart scale — make sure the device that's running the Fitbit app is connected to Wi-Fi.

TIP

Wait, what if the device that's running the Fitbit app doesn't have Bluetooth? That's a drag, but you're not out of luck. You need to purchase Fitbit's wireless sync dongle, which is available from www.fitbit.com/store#accessories.

There are two ways to get started:

» If you're setting up your first Fitbit device, you should have completed the first part of the setup process, as I discussed in the preceding section.

» If you're configuring another Fitbit device, note that you can connect to only one Bluetooth-based device at a time, so connecting to a second device will replace the original device in your account. If that's cool with you, use the Fitbit app to launch the setup process by selecting the Dashboard tab, selecting the Account icon in the top-right corner of the app window, and then selecting Set Up a Device. In the device list displayed by the Fitbit app, select the device you're setting up and then select a device subtype, if asked. Select Set Up (or Set Up Your *Device*) or, if you're setting up a second device that will replace the original, select Switch to *Device*. Select I Agree when the terms and policies show up.

Now follow these steps:

1. **For most Fitbit devices, you first see one or more screens that explain the basic device components and charging instructions. Select Next on each screen.**

    After the introductory formalities, the Fitbit app uses Bluetooth to look for your Fitbit device. Make sure your Fitbit device and your app device are within 33 feet of each other. When the app locates your Fitbit device, the app displays a four-digit number of the device screen.

2. **In the Fitbit app, enter the four-digit code that you see on the Fitbit device display.**

    The Fitbit app device asks whether you want to allow the device to connect to — that is, *pair* with — the Fitbit app.

3. **Select Pair (iOS) or Allow (Windows 10).**

4. **For Fitbit devices that use Wi-Fi, select Next to display a list of nearby Wi-Fi networks. Select your Wi-Fi network, enter the network password, and then select Connect (iOS) or OK (Android).**

    At this point, the Fitbit app checks to see if your Fitbit device is using the latest software. If not, the app will prompt you to update the device:

- For devices connected to Wi-Fi, the update occurs over the Wi-Fi network's internet connection.

- For all other devices, the update occurs over the Internet connection of the device running the Fitbit app. This process requires a Bluetooth connection between the devices, so make sure the devices are close to each other.

5. **Select Update *Device* (iOS; where *Device* is the type of Fitbit device you're configuring) or Next (Android or Windows 10) to perform the update.**

   After the update is complete, the rest of the setup process consists of one or more screens that introduce you to your new Fitbit.

6. **Select Next on each screen to run through introduction.**

Removing a Fitbit Device from Your Account

If you sell, give away, or lose your Fitbit device, you need to remove it from your account:

» **Android:** In the Dashboard, tap the Account icon in the top-right corner, tap the device you want to get rid of, and then tap Remove (the trash can icon in the top-right corner). When the app asks you to confirm, tap Unpair.

» **iOS:** In the Dashboard, tap the Account icon in the top-right corner, tap the device you want to get rid of, and then tap Remove This *Device* (where *Device* is the Fitbit device type). When the app asks you to confirm, tap Remove This *Device*.

» **Fitbit.com:** Surf to www.fitbit.com, log in to your account, select View Settings, and then select your Fitbit device. Select Remove This *Device* From Your Account (where *Device* is your Fitbit's device type). When you are asked to confirm, select Remove.

Taking a Tour of the Fitbit App

Before going any further (both literally and figuratively), you should take a minute or three to acquaint yourself with the layout of the Fitbit app land. To get some landmarks in view, Figure 3-4 shows the iPhone version of the app — the Android version is nearly identical — and Figure 3-5 shows the Windows 10 version.

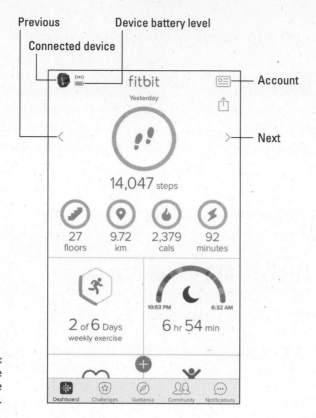

Previous

Connected device

Device battery level

Account

Next

fitbit

Yesterday

14,047 steps

27 floors

9.72 km

2,379 cals

92 minutes

2 of 6 Days
weekly exercise

10:53 PM   6:32 AM

6 hr 54 min

Dashboard   Challenges   Guidance   Community   Notifications

FIGURE 3-4:
The iPhone
version of the
Fitbit app.

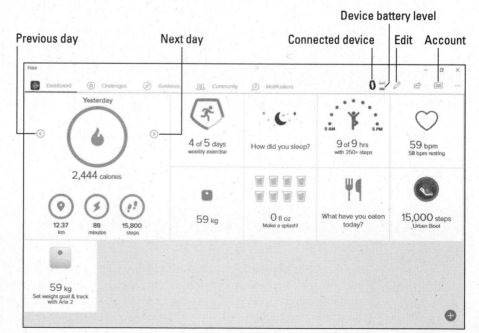

Previous day

Next day

Device battery level

Connected device

Edit

Account

Fitbit

Dashboard   Challenges   Guidance   Community   Notifications

Yesterday

2,444 calories

12.37 km

88 minutes

15,800 steps

4 of 5 days
weekly exercise

How did you sleep?

9 AM   5 PM

9 of 9 hrs
with 250+ steps

59 bpm
58 bpm resting

59 kg

0 fl oz
Make a splash!

What have you eaten
today?

15,000 steps
Urban Boot

59 kg
Set weight goal & track
with Aria 2

FIGURE 3-5:
The Windows 10
version of the
Fitbit app.

As pointed out in both Figures 3-4 and 3-5, the Fitbit app offers the following features:

- » **Fitbit device:** This icon represents your connected Fitbit device. See "Working with Your Fitbit," later in this chapter.

- » **Account:** Tap this icon to access the Account page, which you can use to view and edit your Fitbit profile, set up a family account, add devices, set goals, adjust privacy and security options, and adjust app settings.

- » **Dashboard:** Select this icon to display the Dashboard screen, which displays a summary of the progress of today's health and fitness metrics. Each metric appears in a special rectangle called a *tile*. You can use the Previous Day and Next Day arrows to navigate your historic data.

- » **Challenges:** Select this icon to open the Challenges screen, which you can use to sign up for races and adventures, and compete against family and friends (see Chapter 4).

- » **Guidance:** Select this icon to see the Guidance screen, which gives you access to Fitbit-generated workouts.

- » **Community:** Select this icon to open the Community page, where you can connect with friends, join Fitbit groups, and share your latest health or fitness achievements with other Fitbit users. See Chapter 4 to learn the details.

- » **Notifications:** Select this icon see your most recent notifications from the app. Select the Messages tab to see your latest messages from your Fitbit friends.

Customizing Your Fitbit Account

The Fitbit app offers lots of ways to customize your Fitbit experience to help you get the most out of your tracker and your account. You can configure the dashboard, customize your profile, change app settings, and more.

Configuring the Fitbit app dashboard

When you're using the Fitbit app, you'll spend the bulk of your time obsessing over — er, I mean, *studying* — the metrics to track your progress today and to compare your recent data with past achievements. However, right out of the box, the Dashboard is set up with a generic collection of tiles, some of which might not interest you. If that's the case, it makes sense to simplify your life by customizing your Dashboard to show only the tiles you want to see and to rearrange the tiles to put the most important ones at the top for easy viewing. Just follow these steps:

1. **Select the Dashboard.**

2. **Open the Dashboard for editing:**

   - *Android:* Scroll down to the bottom of the Dashboard screen and tap Edit. The Fitbit app displays a Remove (–) icon in the upper-left corner of each displayed tile and an Add (+) icon in the upper-left corner of each hidden tile.

   - *iOS:* Scroll down to the bottom of the Dashboard screen and tap Edit. The Fitbit app displays a Remove icon (X) icon in the upper-left corner of each displayed tile and an Add (+) icon in the upper-left corner of each hidden tile.

   - *Windows 10:* Select the Edit icon (pencil), which is labeled in Figure 3-5. The Fitbit app displays a Remove (X) icon in the upper-left corner of each displayed tile and an Add (+) icon in the upper-left corner of each hidden tile.

3. **Select the Remove icon (-) for each displayed tile you want to hide.**

4. **Select the Add icon (+) for each hidden tile you want to display.**

5. **To move a tile, drag it to the position you prefer.**

6. **When you're finished, turn off Dashboard editing:**

   - *Android or iOS:* Tap Done at the bottom of the screen.

   - *Windows 10:* Select the Edit icon to turn it off.

Configuring your online Fitbit Dashboard

The Fitbit app's Dashboard is the handiest way to monitor your health and fitness metrics, but what's a numbers nerd to do if she doesn't have the app handy? First, don't panic! Second, calmly check to see if you have a web browser nearby. You do? Good. Now you can get your Fitbit fix by using the online version of the Dashboard.

Surf to www.fitbit.com and then log in to your Fitbit account. You see your Dashboard, which will look similar to the one in Figure 3-6.

Here are the techniques you can use to configure this Dashboard to suit your style:

» To rearrange the tiles, drag any part of a tile to the position you prefer.

» To hide a tile, hover the mouse cursor over the tile, select the Settings icon (gear) that appears just below the tile, select the Remove Tile button (or the trash can icon, if you don't see the button), and then select Remove when Fitbit asks you to confirm.

>> To display a hidden tile, first make sure that you're displaying today's metrics. Select the Menu icon (labeled in Figure 3-6), select the check box beside the tile you want to add, and then select Done.

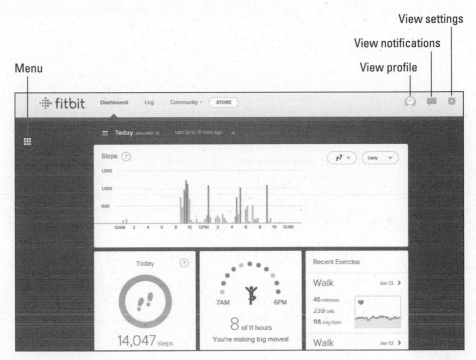

FIGURE 3-6: Log in to Fitbit. com to see your online Dashboard.

Customizing your Fitbit profile

When you first signed up for a Fitbit account, the setup program asked you for some personal info, such as your birthday, weight, and height. Together, these and a few other stats and settings make up your Fitbit profile. To make changes to your existing profile data and to add personal info such as a flattering picture, your home country, and a short description of yourself, follow these steps:

1. **In the Fitbit app, select Dashboard ⇨ Account.**

2. **Select View Your Profile.**

   In the Android app, you don't see the View Your Profile command, so instead tap your name near the top of the Account screen.

3. **Select the camera icon that appears beside the default profile picture, give the app permission to use your device's photos and camera, and then either take a new picture or select an existing picture.**

   You can also choose an image that appears in the header at the top of your profile page by selecting the camera icon that appears beside the default header image.

4. **Select Personal.**

   The app displays the Personal screen, which contains your profile data.

5. **For each piece of info you want to edit, select the info and then make your changes. If you see a Save button, be sure to select it to save your changes.**

To customize your profile online instead of in the app, point your trusty web browser to www.fitbit.com and log in to your account to display the Dashboard. Select View Settings (labeled in Figure 3-6), and then select Settings. You should now see the Personal Info page; if you don't, select Personal Info.

Adjusting Fitbit app settings

As a final configuration chore before getting to the good stuff, you should adjust a few settings for the Fitbit app itself. These settings include the measurement units you prefer (such as miles or kilometers), your time zone, and on what day your week begins.

1. **In the Fitbit app, select Dashboard ⇨ Account.**

2. **Select Advanced Settings.**

   The Advanced Settings screen appears. Figure 3-7 shows the Android version.

3. **To set the time zone:**

WARNING

   Don't adjust the time zone unless you really have to, especially if the new time zone would roll back the time because you'll lose all generated data between now and the new earlier time. A new time zone that rolls the time forward is problematic as well because it creates a gap in your data between now and the new later time.

   - *Android:* Tap the Automatic Time Zone switch to Off, tap Select Time Zone, and then tap the time zone you want to use.

   - *iOS:* Tap the Set Automatically switch to Off, tap Time Zone, and then tap the time zone you want to use.

   - *Windows 10:* Select Time Zone, select the Auto switch to Off, tap Time Zone, and then tap the time zone you want to use.

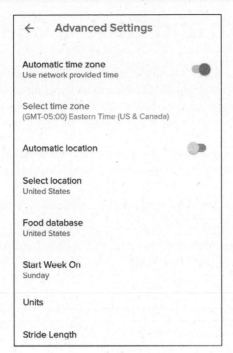

4. **To set your location (that is, your country):**

   • *Android:* Tap the Automatic Location switch to Off, tap Select Location, and then tap your country.

   • *iOS:* Tap Location, tap the Automatic switch to Off, and then tap your country.

   • *Windows 10:* Select Country, select the Auto switch to Off, and then tap your country.

5. **To set the measurement units, select Units, and then select your preferred units for length, weight, and water consumption.**

   In the Android and iOS version of the Fitbit app, you can also select a measurement unit for swimming.

6. **To set the start of the week, select Start Week On and then select either Sunday or Monday.**

The Advanced Settings screen has quite a few other app settings, but I'll hold off covering them here and instead tell you about them in the relevant sections of the book. (For example, I talk about setting the food database in Chapter 10.)

Setting Your Health and Fitness Goals

Every health and fitness expert worthy of the name will tell you that good intentions aren't worth the proverbial hill of beans unless those intentions are anchored by realistic and measurable goals. Anyone can learn to shoot an arrow, but you know you're getting better at it only if you aim for the bull's-eye.

What kinds of goals should you set? The answer depends on what you're trying to accomplish with your Fitbit. Following are six general categories of goals:

>> **Activity:** The number of steps you take and the number of minutes you're active each day

>> **Exercise:** The number of days you exercise, that is, walk, run, bike, play sports, or perform some other aerobic exercise

>> **Weight:** The body weight you're shooting for

>> **Calories:** The number of calories you consume each day

>> **Water:** The number of glasses of water you drink each day

>> **Sleep:** The number of hours you sleep each night

Setting your initial goals

The folks at Fitbit know the importance of goals, so the Fitbit app prompts you at the beginning to set some health and fitness targets. Here's the procedure to follow:

1. **Launch the goal-setting process:**

   • *Android:* Tap the Let Us Help You Set Some Goals message.

   • *iOS or Windows 10:* Select the Set Goals button.

2. **In the initial screen, select Let's Go.**

   As shown in Figure 3-8, the Fitbit app displays a list of goals, such as Manage My Weight and Up My Daily Steps and Activity.

3. **Select the goal that means the most to you or is the best fit.**

   The app asks why that goal is important to you and offers several answers.

4. **Select an answer.**

   The app presents several statements and asks which of them is most true about your health and fitness.

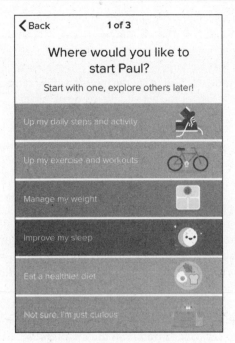

FIGURE 3-8:
The Fitbit app asks you to select an initial goal.

Where would you like to start Paul?

Start with one, explore others later!

Up my daily steps and activity

Up my exercise and workouts

Manage my weight

Improve my sleep

Eat a healthier diet

Not sure. I'm just curious

5. **Select the statement that most accurately or strongly reflects how you feel.**

   The app lets you know that it has three recommended goals based on your answers.

6. **Select Take a Look.**

   The app shows you the first goal. To describe this goal as "recommended" is disingenuous, to say the least, because the app offers no way to *not* choose this goal!

7. **Adjust the goal, as needed (for example, by increasing or decreasing the number of steps), and then select Make This My Goal.**

   The app displays several more goals and asks you to choose two. Fortunately, these goals are optional, so you can choose as many or as few as you like.

8. **Select each goal you want to add, and then select Let's Do This.**

9. **For each goal you selected, adjust the goal's target value as needed and then select Make This My Goal.**

   Examples of target values include the number of minutes of activity each day and the number of days of exercise each week. When you're finished, the app displays a summary of your goals.

When setting up the specifics of your goals, be realistic. If you make your goals too ambitious, you might get discouraged if you fall short each time. On the other hand, don't make your targets too easy, or you might get bored. If you're just starting out, it's probably best to set the targets a little on the easy side; you can make them harder as you get into the swing of things.

10. **Select Looks Good.**

The app sets your goals, and you can track your progress using the Goals section of the app's Account page.

Adjusting your goals

As you get healthier and more fit, you'll want to nudge up your goal targets to keep improving and stay motivated. Similarly, if you find that your initial goals are too hard or too easy, you should adjust your targets accordingly so that you have proper goals to shoot for.

I go into more details about specific goals in the relevant sections of the book. If you're not sure where to set your targets, see the chapters for activity, sleep, and so on in Part 2.

Here are the steps to follow to adjust your goal values:

1. **In the Fitbit app, select Dashboard ⇨ Account.**

2. **In the Goals section, select Activity to open the Activity Goals screen (see Figure 3-9). For each metric, tap the activity and then enter a new value.**

In the Android or iOS app, when you're finished, tap Back to return to the Account screen.

‹ Account Activity Goals	
Daily Activity	
Steps	10,000 steps
Distance	8.05 km
Calories Burned	2,268 cals
Active Minutes	40 minutes
Floors Climbed	10 floors
Hourly Activity Goal	9 hr/day

FIGURE 3-9: Set activity targets such as your daily steps, distance, and active minutes.

3. **In the Goals section, select Exercise to open the Exercise Goals screen. Select the Weekly Exercise Goals value, and then select the number of days of exercise you want to shoot for each week. In the Android app, tap Save.**

   In the Android or iOS app, when you're done, tap Back until you return to the Account screen.

4. **In the Goals section, select Nutrition & Body to open the Nutrition & Body Goals screen. For each metric, select the goal and enter the new value.**

   In the Android or iOS app, when you're done, tap Back until you return to the Account screen.

5. **In the Goals section, select Sleep to open the Sleep Goals screen. Select the Time Asleep goal, and then follow the onscreen instructions.**

   For details, see Chapter 6.

   In the Android or iOS app, when you're done, tap Back until you return to the Account screen.

Working with Your Fitbit

I open this chapter by cautioning you to not just slap your new Fitbit onto your wrist and head out the door. If you heeded that advice, wow, thanks! Your patience will now be rewarded because it's time for your wrist and your Fitbit to get acquainted. The rest of this chapter takes you through a few useful techniques and tips for getting you and your Fitbit on familiar terms.

Setting your Fitbit's wrist placement

You wear your Fitbit on your wrist, but does it matter which wrist you use? Nope, not at all, as along as the Fitbit app knows two things: which wrist you're using and which is your dominant hand (also known as your *handedness*). These tidbits are needed because Fitbit alters its tracking slightly if you're using your dominant hand, which not only tends to get more overall use during the day but is also used for potentially tracker-confounding activities such as throwing a ball and giving a high five.

TIP

If you have the Alta HR, Charge 3, Inspire HR, Ionic, Versa, or another Fitbit device that monitors heart rate, position the tracker about a finger-width above your wrist bone for the most accurate heart rate readings. During exercise, shift the tracker to about three finger-widths above the wrist bone — and wear the device slightly tighter than usual — to keep the heart rate readings accurate.

You specified which wrist you're using for your Fitbit during setup, but if you change wrists or if you want to make sure Fitbit is using the correct handedness value for you, following these steps:

1. **In the Fitbit app, select Dashboard ⇨ Account.**

2. **Select your Fitbit device.**

3. **Use the Wrist setting to choose the wrist on which you're wearing your Fitbit: Left or Right.**

4. **Tell Fitbit which is your dominant hand:**

   - **Ace, Alta, or Alta HR:** Use the Handedness setting to specify your handedness: Righty (that is, your right hand is dominant) or Lefty (your left hand is dominant).

   - **Charge 3, Flex 2, Inspire, Inspire HR, Ionic, or Versa:** Use the Wrist Placement setting (or just Wrist on the Flex 2) to specify which wrist you're using for your Fitbit: Dominant or Non-Dominant.

Navigating your Fitbit's interface

Whether you want to see the current time, view your daily health and fitness stats, or crank up an app, you need to know how to wake and navigate your Fitbit. Here are the basics:

» **Waking the screen automatically:** When the Quick View or Screen Wake feature is on (the name depends on the Fitbit), you can wake your Fitbit device by turning your wrist towards you. To control the Quick View or Screen Wake feature:

   - *Ace, Alta, or Alta HR:* In the Fitbit app, select Dashboard ⇨ Account, select your Fitbit device, and then toggle the Quick View switch On or Off.

   - *Charge 3, Ionic, Inspire, Inspire HR, or Versa:* Press and hold down the Back button (see the next section), and then tap Screen Wake to toggle this setting between Auto (the feature is on) and Manual (the feature is off).

» **Waking the screen manually:** Double-tap the screen. If you have the Ace, Alta, Alta HR, or Flex 2, it's best to double-tap the screen near the bottom edge (or the top edge) where it meets the wristband.

» **Navigating the screen:** After your Fitbit is awake, how you navigate the screen depends on the device:

- *Ace, Alta, or Alta HR:* Tap the display to jump to the next screen of your daily stats.

- *Charge 3, Ionic, Inspire, Inspire HR, or Versa:* Swipe up or down to navigate the screen vertically and view your daily stats; swipe left or right to navigate the screen horizontally and access your device's apps.

Pushing your Fitbit's buttons

Fitbit devices such as the Ace, Alta, and Alta HR have a pleasingly simple design consisting of a tappable display that connects to a wristband. But newer Fitbits — particularly the Inspire wristband and the Ionic and Versa watches — come with one or more buttons that you can press or hold down to navigate the device screen. Here's a quick look at these buttons, where they're located, and what you can do with them:

» **Charge 3, Inspire, or Inspire HR:** These devices have a single button on the left side of the display, as shown in Figure 3-10. You can press this button to wake the device and put it to sleep. Also, pressing this button while the device is awake takes you back to the previous level in the hierarchy. Press and hold down on the button for about two seconds to access the device's quick settings.

Back

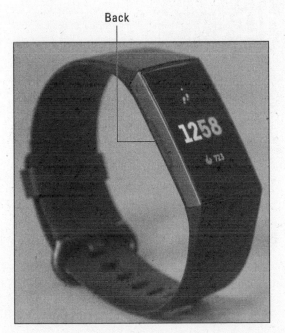

FIGURE 3-10:
The Fitbit Charge 3 tracker has a single button.

>> **Ionic and Versa:** These devices have three buttons: one on the left side of the display and two on the right, as shown in Figure 3-11:

- *Back:* Press this button to wake and sleep the device. Pressing this button when the device is awake takes you back to the previous level in the hierarchy. Press and hold down the button for about two seconds to access the device's quick settings.

- *Top:* Press this button to wake the device. Pressing this button when the clock is displayed opens the app located in the top-left corner of the first app screen (see "Using apps on your Fitbit watch," later in this chapter). You can also press and hold down the button for about two seconds to access the device's notifications.

- *Bottom:* Press this button to wake the device. Pressing this button when the clock is displayed opens the app located in the bottom-left corner of the first app screen.

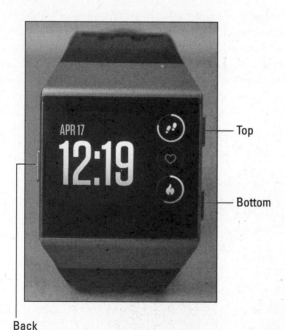

FIGURE 3-11:
The Fitbit Ionic watch has three buttons.

Getting app notifications on your Fitbit

If your Fitbit is close enough to your phone, tablet, or computer for a Bluetooth connection, you can receive notifications for events such as an incoming call or text message, or a calendar alert. Getting notifications on your tracker can be handy because if you can't see the screen of your other device, a quick glance at your wrist lets you know what's going on. If you miss a notification, swipe down from the top of the device screen to see past notifications.

Customizing notifications

To set up which apps can send notifications to your Fitbit and to set a few other notification-related options, follow these steps:

1. **In the Fitbit app, select Dashboard ⇨ Account.**

2. **Select your Fitbit device.**

3. **Select Notifications.**

4. **If you see a message asking you to give Fitbit permission to make and manage phone calls, contacts, and text message, select Allow in each case.**

   Figure 3-12 shows the Android version of the Notifications screen that appears.

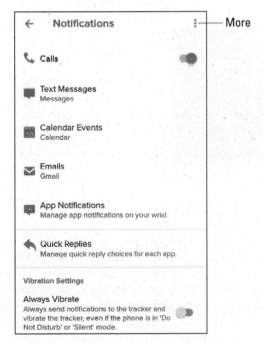

FIGURE 3-12: You can customize Fitbit notifications.

5. **Use the Calls, Text Messages, and Calendar Events settings to enable, configure, or disable notifications for these events.**

   In the Android app, you can also set up notifications for Emails.

6. **To add notifications for other apps on your Android or iOS device, tap App Notifications and then select which apps you want to use.**

7. **In the Android app, tap Quick Replies to set up reply shortcuts for each app currently displaying notifications on your Fitbit.**

8. **In the Android app, if you want to receive notifications even if your device is in Do Not Disturb mode or Silent mode, tap the Always Vibrate switch to On.**

Disabling notifications

In the Android app, you can disable all notifications by tapping the More icon (labeled in Figure 3-12) and then tapping Disable Notifications. In the Charge 3, Ionic, Inspire, Inspire HR, or Versa, you can disable notifications by pressing and holding down the device's Back button to display the quick settings, and then tapping the Notifications setting to Off, as shown in Figure 3-13.

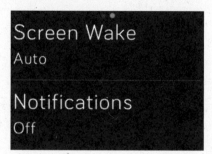

FIGURE 3-13:
In the device's quick settings, you can tap Notifications to Off.

Syncing your Fitbit

Your Fitbit device spends its day gathering info about your activities and body states, such as your heart rate. How does all that data get from your Fitbit to the Fitbit app? In a behind-the-scenes process called *syncing*, the device and the app connect to each other and the device passes along its latest hoard of data (and the app might send the device some stuff, too, such as updated settings or personal data).

Fortunately, you don't have to worry about syncing most of the time because it's set up by default to happen automatically, as follows:

>> Every time you open the Fitbit app, as long as the app and the device are paired.

>> Periodically throughout the day, as long as the app device and the Fitbit device are within range and you have the All-Day Sync option turned on. To check the latter, open the Fitbit app's Dashboard, select the Account icon (labeled in Figures 3-4 and 3-5), select your Fitbit device, and then make sure the All-Day Sync switch is set to On.

If you don't think you're seeing the latest data in your Dashboard, you can make sure by syncing your Fitbit device manually. Make sure the Fitbit app device and the Fitbit device are within about 20 feet of each other, and then use the technique appropriate to your device's operating system:

>> **Android or iOS:** Display the Dashboard, pull down the screen until you see the Release to Sync message, and then release the screen. Alternatively, tap the Fitbit device icon and then tap Sync Now.

>> **Windows 10:** Display the Dashboard, select the Fitbit device icon (labeled in Figure 3-4) and then select the Sync icon, shown in Figure 3-14. Alternatively, select the Account icon, select your Fitbit device, and then select Sync Now.

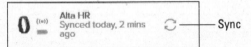

Using apps on your Fitbit watch

Some Fitbit devices — notably the Ionic and Versa watches and the Charge 3 tracker — can run *apps* (or *applications*), which are mini-programs that perform specific tasks. Six default apps are installed on these devices:

>> **Alarms:** Set up silent alarms that trigger at a time and day you specify. See Chapter 11.

>> **Exercise:** Tell Fitbit that you're performing a specific exercise session, such as a run or a weight workout. See Chapter 9.

>> **Relax:** Perform guided deep-breathing for a specified time. See Chapter 11.

>> **Settings:** Display settings and options for customizing the device.

>> **Timers:** Set a countdown timer (discussed in Chapter 11) or use a stopwatch to time an event.

>> **Weather:** Display the current weather in your area.

The Ionic and Versa watches have even more apps, including a few apps for connecting to third-party services such as Deezer, Strava, and Starbucks (see Chapter 14). In addition, the following apps help you get more out of your Fitbit:

>> **Coach:** Access guided video workouts.

>> **Music:** Play music that you've stored on your watch, as described in Chapter 14.

>> **Tips:** Display a series of quick tips to help you learn more about your device.

>> **Today:** Peruse your steps, heart rate, and other daily metrics. With the clock displayed, swipe up from the bottom of the screen to launch the Today app.

>> **Wallet:** Use Fitbit Pay to make contactless payments.

That's awesome, for sure, but you'll no doubt be amazed to learn that there are *thousands* more apps available and you can install any of them on your Ionic or Versa watch (alas, these extra apps can't be installed on the Charge 3).

Installing an app

Follow these steps to install an app:

1. **In the Fitbit app, select Dashboard ➪ Account, and then select your Fitbit device.**

2. **Select Apps.**

3. **Select the All Apps tab.**

4. **Locate an app that looks interesting or useful, and select Install.**

5. **If the app requests permissions, select the check box for each permission and then select Install.**

    The Fitbit app installs the app and adds it to the watch the next time it performs a sync.

Arranging apps

If you have an Ionic or Versa watch, you can change the order of the apps. This feature is useful if you use two apps most of the time: When the clock is displayed, pressing the Top button (refer to Figure 3-11) automatically opens the app that appears in the top-left corner of the first app screen, and pressing the Bottom button automatically opens the app that appears in the bottom-left corner of the first app screen.

To change the order of the app icons, follow these steps:

1. **Turn on the watch and make sure the clock is displayed.**

2. **Swipe left until you get to the app screen you want to organize.**

3. **Press and hold down on the icon of the app you want to move.**

   The watch vibrates briefly and the app names disappear.

4. **Drag the app icon to the location you want.**

   To navigate to the previous or next app screen, drag the icon to the left or right edge of the screen, respectively.

5. **Release the icon.**

   Your Fitbit device places the app into the new position and rearranges the other app icons accordingly.

Uninstalling an app

If an app you installed has become bothersome or boring, get rid of it by following these steps:

1. **In the Fitbit app, select Dashboard ⇨ Account, and then select your Fitbit device.**

2. **Select Apps.**

3. **Select the My Apps tab.**

4. **Select Remove.**

   The Fitbit app uninstalls the app. Note that if you don't see the Remove button, it means you can't uninstall the app (which is the case for many default apps, such as Exercise and Settings).

IN THIS CHAPTER

» **Choosing a cool name for your public posts**

» **Connecting with Fitbit friends**

» **Setting up a Fitbit account for family members**

» **Joining, viewing, and participating in Fitbit groups**

» **Posting workouts, badges, and other achievements to the Fitbit community**

Chapter **4**

Getting Social

Tracking your steps, exercise, heart rate, weight, and food and water consumption seems like an inherently solitary business. It's not called *self*-tracking for nothing. If you want to keep all that data to yourself, that's fine. However, countless studies have shown that adding a social component to your health and fitness regime can greatly increase your chances of both sticking to that regime and achieving whatever goals you've set for yourself. If you announce to selected friends and family members that you want to lose 20 pounds, knowing that other people are aware of your goal makes you more motivated to achieve it. If your sibling makes it known that she did 11,000 steps yesterday, that might fire you up to do 12,000 today.

The folks at Fitbit are well aware of the significant benefits that accrue when you make your self-tracking public, so they've built tons of social features into the Fitbit app. In this chapter, you discover these features and learn how they can help you start up, stick with, and succeed at a health and fitness program.

Setting a Fitbit Username

Before you start sharing your self-tracking with others, you need to decide on a moniker that will identify you to the Fitbit community. Most folks use their first name and last initial, but you can also create a *username*, which is a kind of nickname. If you want maximum privacy while still doing the social thing, a username is the way to go.

Adding a username to your account

Here are the steps to follow to add a username to your Fitbit account:

1. **In the Fitbit app, select Dashboard ⇨ Account.**

2. **Select View Your Profile.**

   The Android app doesn't display the View Your Profile text, so tap your name near the top of the Account screen.

3. **If you see the Welcome to Community introduction, select Next until you reach the last screen, then select Done.**

4. **Select Personal.**

5. **Select Display Name.**

   The Display Name screen appears. Figure 4-1 shows the iPhone version of this screen.

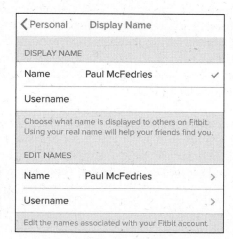

FIGURE 4-1:
The iPhone version of the Display Name screen.

6. **Specify the username you want to add:**

   • *Android or iOS:* In the Edit Names section, tap Username, enter the username you want to add, and then tap Save.

   • *Windows 10:* Enter the username you want to add in the Username text box.

   The username you enter can contain only letters, numbers, and hyphens (-), and it can be no more than 20 characters long.

7. **Select Save.**

   Fitbit reminds you that you can change your name every sixty days.

8. **Select OK (Android or iOS) or Yes (Windows 10).**

   The Fitbit app saves your username. If, instead, you see a message telling you the username is already taken, repeat Steps 65 through 8 to try again.

Setting your username as your display name

Your Fitbit *display name* is the name that appears in your group posts, challenges, and other social activities. By default, Fitbit uses your first name and last initial as your display name. To control whether Fitbit uses your name or your username for display purposes, follow these steps.

1. **In the Fitbit app, select Dashboard ⇨ Account.**

2. **Select View Your Profile.**

   The Android app doesn't display the View Your Profile text, so tap your name near the top of the Account screen.

3. **Select Personal.**

4. **Select Display Name.**

5. **Specify which name you want to use as your display name:**

   • *Android or iOS:* In the Display Name section, tap either Name or Username.

   • *Windows 10:* In the Display As section, select either Name or User Name and then select Save.

   The Fitbit app saves your display name.

Connecting with Friends

You can take your Fitbit experience up a notch by connecting with people you know who are also on Fitbit. After you add someone as a friend, you can do the following:

>> See where you rank with respect to the total steps taken over the past week

>> See that person's latest activities

>> Exchange encouraging (or taunting) messages

>> Challenge that person to a competition

>> Share your latest Fitbit achievements

The Fitbit app gives you four ways to add friends to your Fitbit social circle:

>> **Contacts:** The Fitbit app scours your device contacts, looking for those who have Fitbit accounts.

>> **Facebook:** The Fitbit app digs through your Facebook friends to see who does the Fitbit thing.

>> **Email:** You enter the email address of a person who you know has a Fitbit account.

>> **Username:** You enter the username of a person who you know has a Fitbit account.

I discuss the details of each method in this section.

Sending a friend request to your contacts

You might be leery of letting Fitbit rummage around in your contacts, but the company promises not to send anything to a contact without your permission. If that seems reasonable, you need to give the Fitbit app permission to access your contacts and then send your request:

1. **In the Fitbit app, select Community.**

2. **Select the Friends tab.**

   The Friends tab is where the Fitbit app will eventually list all your friends, ranked in descending order of total steps taken over the past week. For now, it's either empty or you see just yourself, as shown in the Android version in Figure 4-2.

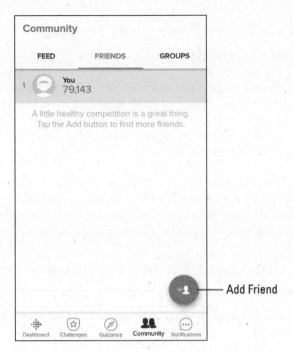

Community

FEED   FRIENDS   GROUPS

1   You
      79,143

A little healthy competition is a great thing.
Tap the Add button to find more friends.

+1 ——— Add Friend

Dashboard   Challenges   Guidance   Community   Notifications

FIGURE 4-2:
The Android
version of the
Friends tab.

3. **Select the Add Friend icon (labeled in Figure 4-2).**

4. **Select the Contacts tab.**

5. **Give Fitbit permission to access your contacts:**

   - *Android:* Tap Enable, and when your Android asks you to confirm, tap Allow.

   - *iOS:* Tap Connect Contacts, and when iOS asks you to confirm, tap OK.

   - *Windows 10:* Select Open Settings to run the Settings app, which automatically displays the Contacts tab of the Privacy page. Select Change, turn on the Contacts Access for This Device switch, and then turn on the Fitbit switch. Restart the Fitbit app, repeat Steps 1 through 4, and then skip to Step 6. (Note that the switch is green when it's on.)

   The Fitbit app's Contacts tab now displays two lists. At the top you see *X* Contacts with Fitbit, where *X* is the number of people the Fitbit app found in your contacts who have a Fitbit account. Below that list you see the Contacts without Fitbit list.

6. **Select the Add Friend icon beside the contact you want to add.**

   The Add Friend icon turns into a clock icon, indicating that the app is waiting for the other person to accept (or — horrors! — reject) your friend request.

Sending a friend request to your Facebook friends

If you know some people on Facebook who rock a Fitbit, it might be easier to add them as Fitbit friends by letting the Fitbit app scour your Facebook connections. Fitbit claims that they won't reach out to any Facebook friend without asking you first, so why not? Before this can happen, you have to give the Fitbit app permission to access your Facebook account.

In the sections that follow, you give Fitbit permission to access your Facebook account. If, down the road, you want to revoke that permission, you have to do it on the Facebook site. Log in to your Facebook account, select Settings ⇨ Apps and Websites, select the Fitbit check box, and then select Remove.

Using the Fitbit app to send a Facebook friend request

Here are the steps to follow to ship out a request to a Facebook friend by using the Fitbit app:

1. **Select Community.**

2. **Select the Friends tab.**

3. **Select the Add Friend icon (labeled in Figure 4-2).**

4. **Select the Facebook tab.**

5. **Select Connect Facebook.**

    The app prompts you to log in to your Facebook account.

6. **Enter your Facebook login credentials, and then select Log In.**

    A screen shows you what Facebook permissions you're giving to the Fitbit app.

7. **Select Continue as *Name*, where *Name* is your first name.**

    The Fitbit app connects to your Facebook account and examines your friends to see which of them have Fitbit accounts.

    The Fitbit app's Facebook tab now displays a list of your Facebook friends who have a Fitbit account.

8. **Select the Add Friend icon beside the Facebook friend you want to add.**

    The Add Friend icon turns into a clock icon, indicating that the app is waiting for the other person to accept (or summarily reject) your friend request.

Using Fitbit.com to send a Facebook friend request

Here are the steps to follow to send a request to a Facebook friend by using Fitbit.com:

1. **Surf to www.fitbit.com and log in to your account.**

2. **In the Friends tile, select Connect Facebook.**

   Fitbit prompts you to log in to your Facebook account.

3. **Enter your Facebook login credentials, and then select Log In.**

   A screen shows you what Facebook permissions you're giving to the Fitbit app.

4. **Select Continue as *Name*, where *Name* is your first name.**

   Fitbit connects to your Facebook account. After a few moments, the Friends tile displays a list of your Facebook friends who have a Fitbit account.

5. **Select the Add Friend button beside the person you want to add.**

   By default, Fitbit displays only a few Facebook friends in the Friends tile. To see the rest of your Fitbit-connected Facebook friends, hover the mouse pointer over the Friends tile, select See More (or surf to www.fitbit.com/friends), and then select the Show All link that appears above your Facebook friends list (which Fitbit labels May We Suggest).

   The Add Friend icon turns into a clock icon, indicating that Fitbit is waiting for the other person to accept (or — say it isn't so — reject) your friend request.

Sending a friend request by email

If you know the email address of a person's Fitbit account, you can send a friend request to that email address.

Using the Fitbit app to send an email friend request

Here are the steps to follow to send an email friend request by using the Fitbit app:

1. **In the Fitbit app, select Community.**

2. **Select the Friends tab.**

3. **Select the Add Friend icon (labeled in Figure 4-2).**

4. **Select the Email tab.**

5. **Enter the person's email address.**

   When the address is complete, the Fitbit app displays a friend request for that person.

6. **Select the Add Friend icon beside the friend request.**

   The Add Friend icon turns into a clock icon, indicating that the app is waiting for the other person to accept (or — boo! — reject) your friend request.

Using Fitbit.com to send an email friend request

Here are the steps to follow to send one or more email friend requests using Fitbit.com:

1. **Surf to www.fitbit.com and log in to your account.**

2. **In the Friends tile, select Invite Friends.**

   If you've already connected your Facebook account to Fitbit, you won't see the Invite Friends link. Instead, hover your mouse pointer over the Friends tile, select Find Friends (or open www.fitbit.com/friends), and then select Invite by Email.

   Fitbit displays the Invite Friends by Email window.

3. **In the Email Addresses text box, enter an email address for each person you want to invite.**

   When you complete an address, type a space or a comma or press tab to complete the address and move to the next one.

   Fitbit displays a sneak peek of your friend request in the Message Preview pane.

4. **When you've entered all your addresses, select Send Invitation.**

   Fitbit ships out your friend requests.

Sending a friend request by using a Fitbit username

If you know a person's Fitbit username, follow these steps to send a friend request to that person:

1. **In the Fitbit app, select Community.**

2. **Select the Friends tab.**

3. **Select the Add Friend icon (labeled in Figure 4-2).**

4. **Select the Username tab.**

5. **Enter the person's username.**

   When the username is complete, the Fitbit app displays a friend request for that person.

6. **Select the Add Friend icon beside the friend request.**

   The Add Friend icon turns into a clock icon, indicating that the app is waiting for the other person to accept (or ungratefully reject) your friend request.

Handling a friend request

When a friend request comes in through Fitbit, one of the following occurs:

» **Android or Windows 10:** You see a notification onscreen similar to the one shown in Figure 4-3, left. Select View to open the request.

» **iOS:** You see a badge on the Fitbit app's Notifications icon, as shown in Figure 4-3, right. Tap Notifications, tap Messages if it isn't already displayed, and then tap the request.

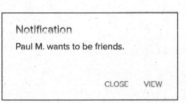

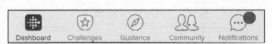

You might receive a friend request also by email or Facebook. From here, you can either select Accept Friend to connect with the sender, or select Ignore to reject the request, as shown in Figure 4-4. An email friend request doesn't have an Ignore option; instead, just delete the message and move on with your life.

Cheering or taunting a friend

After you have one or more friends connected to your Fitbit account, the real fun can begin. I speak, of course, of taunting any friend who has fewer steps than you. To even out your karma, you can also cheer a friend whose step count surpasses yours.

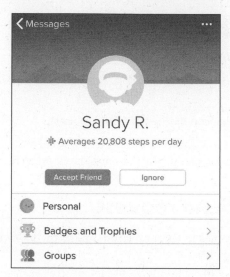

FIGURE 4-4:
Select Accept
Friend to
welcome your
new Fitbit
acquaintance.

Using the Fitbit app to send a cheer or taunt

Here are the steps to follow to send a cheer or taunt to a friend by using the Fitbit app:

1. **Select Community.**

2. **Select the Friends tab.**

3. **Select the friend you want to taunt or cheer.**

    Fitbit displays the friend's profile, as shown in Figure 4-5.

4. **Select the Cheer or the Taunt icon.**

    In the Windows 10 app, these icons appear unlabeled at the bottom of the screen.

Using Fitbit.com to send a cheer or taunt

Here are the steps to follow to send a cheer or taunt to a friend online by using Fitbit.com:

1. **Surf to www.fitbit.com and log in to your account.**

2. **In the Friends tile, hover the mouse pointer over the friend you want to cheer or taunt.**

    Fitbit displays three icons under the friend's name, as shown in Figure 4-6.

3. **Select the Cheer or the Taunt icon.**

    Fitbit sends the cheer or taunt to your friend.

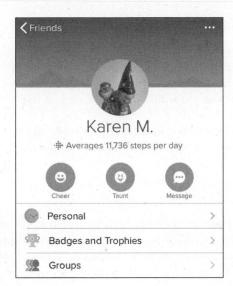

FIGURE 4-5:
To send a cheer
or taunt, first
display the
friend's profile.

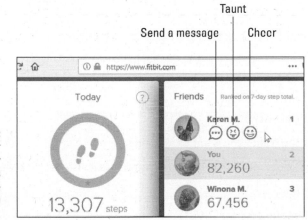

FIGURE 4-6:
Hover your
mouse pointer
over a friend's
icon to see the
Taunt and
Cheer Icons.

Receiving a cheer or taunt

The cheer the friend receives resembles the one shown in Figure 4-7, left, which is the Android version. If you sent a taunt, instead, the Windows 10 version of the message resembles the one shown in Figure 4-7, right.

FIGURE 4-7:
A received
cheer in Android
(left) and a
received taunt
in Windows 10
(right).

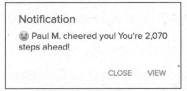

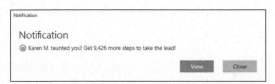

For the iOS version of the Fitbit app, a badge appears on the Notifications icon and, when the person taps Notifications, the cheer or taunt appears in the Notifications tab. If you're logged in to Fitbit.com, select the View Notifications icon (which I point out in Chapter 3). On your Charge 3, Inspire, Ionic, or Versa, wake up the device and then swipe down from the top of the screen.

TIP

If you have an Ionic or Versa watch, you can display your recent messages also by pressing and holding down on the Top button (see Chapter 3).

Messaging a friend

When sending a simple cheer or taunt just won't cut it, banter-wise, you can step up your game by sending a message to a friend. You can compose messages up to 180 characters long. That's even less than Twitter now allows, so you (probably) won't be getting into complex or detailed discussions about training methodology or health science. That's fine, because Fitbit messages are meant to be simple and quick.

Using the Fitbit app to send a message

Follow these steps to send a message by using the Fitbit app:

1. **Select Community.**

2. **Select the Friends tab.**

3. **Select the friend you want to message.**

   Fitbit displays the friend's profile, as shown previously in Figure 4-5.

4. **Select Message.**

   The Fitbit app opens the Message to *Friend* screen, where *Friend* is the name of your friend.

5. **In the large text box, enter your message.**

6. **Select Send.**

   The Fitbit app sends your message to your friend.

Using Fitbit.com to send a message

Here are the steps required to send a message online by using Fitbit.com:

1. **Surf to** www.fitbit.com **and log in to your account.**

2. **In the Friends tile, hover the mouse pointer over the friend you want to message.**

3. **Select the Send a Message icon (labeled in Figure 4-6).**

   Fitbit displays a pop-up window named Message to *Friend*, where *Friend* is the name of the person you're messaging.

4. **In the large text box, enter your message.**

5. **Select Send.**

   Fitbit tosses the message to your friend.

Viewing and replying to a received message

To view a message you received, use any of the following techniques:

TIP

>> **Fitbit device:** On your Charge 3, Inspire, Ionic, or Versa, wake up the device and then swipe down from the top of the screen.

   If you have an Ionic or Versa watch, you can display your recent messages also by pressing and holding down on the Top button (see Chapter 3).

>> **Fitbit app:** Select Notifications ➪ Messages.

>> **Fitbit.com:** Select the Notifications icon.

Here's how to reply to a message:

>> **Fitbit app:** Select the message, enter your reply, and then select Send.

>> **Fitbit.com:** Select the message's Reply link, enter your reply, and then select Send.

Challenging friends

One of the goals of connecting with friends on Fitbit is motivation. The thinking is that if you see a friend putting up big daily step numbers and posting workouts regularly, you'll get fired up to keep your own activity level high (particularly if that friend stoops to taunting you about your relatively puny Fitbit stats).

Another great way to crank up your motivation is to invite a friend to participate in a Fitbit challenge. A *challenge* is a step-based competition to see who can take the most steps during a specified time. For example, in the Weekend Warrior challenge, you compete with up to nine friends to see who can take the most steps Saturday and Sunday. A similar challenge is Workweek Hustle, where you and up to nine Fitbit pals battle to see who can take the most paces Monday through Friday.

Inviting Fitbit friends to a challenge

Follow these steps to invite one or more friends to a challenge:

1. **In the Fitbit app, select Community.**

2. **In the Challenges section, select the challenge you want to start.**

   If you don't see the challenge you want, select the See All link to view the full list of challenges.

   Fitbit displays an overview of the challenge (Figure 4-8 shows an example), which includes the number of participants (between two and ten in the Weekend Warrior example) and the number of days (two in the Weekend Warrior challenge).

   Each challenge has one or more Start buttons, the name (or names) of which will vary depending on the challenge. For example, all the one-day challenges have both a Start Now button and a Start Tomorrow button; the Weekend Warrior challenge has a single Start Saturday button (unless today is Saturday, in which case you see Start Now and Start Next Saturday buttons).

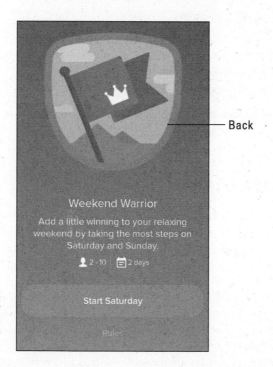

Back

Weekend Warrior

Add a little winning to your relaxing weekend by taking the most steps on Saturday and Sunday.

👤 2 - 10   📅 2 days

Start Saturday

Rules

FIGURE 4-8:
The overview screen of the Weekend Warrior challenge.

3. **Set up the challenge:**

- *Android:* Tap the Start button you want to use, tap the Friends tab, select the check box beside each friend you want to invite to the challenge, and then tap Start Challenge.

- *iOS:* Tap the Start button you want to use, tap the Friends tab, select the check box beside each friend you want to invite to the challenge, and then tap Start.

- *Windows 10:* Select the Friends tab, select the Add icon (+) beside each friend you want to invite to the challenge, and then select the Start button you want to use.

Fitbit sends out the challenge invitations.

Handling a challenge request

When a challenge request comes in through Fitbit, one of the following occurs:

>> **Android or Windows 10:** You see a notification onscreen similar to the one shown in Figure 4-9, left. Select View to open the request and then select either Join the Challenge (Android) or Join Challenge (Windows 10).

>> **iOS:** You see a badge on the Fitbit app's Challenges icon, as shown in Figure 4-9, right. Tap Challenges, tap the invitation, and then tap Join the Challenge.

FIGURE 4-9:
A challenge
request on the
Android (left) and
in iOS (right).

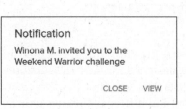

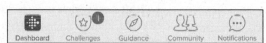

Posting a message to your friends

Got a fine Dashboard going today? Did you hammer a particularly good workout yesterday? If you've done something noteworthy, why not share it with your friends? To do that, follow these steps to post a message:

1. **In the Fitbit app, select Community.**

2. **Select the Feed tab.**

3. **Select the What Are You Up To? text box.**

   Fitbit open the Compose screen, which includes both a text box for a message and several buttons for sharing achievements.

4. **In the What Are You Up To? text box, type a message.**

5. **To share an achievement, tap the corresponding button, and then use the screen that appears to select the specific achievement you want to share.**

6. **If the achievement has display options, select the options you want to use.**

   For example, with a walk or run you can display the exercise heart rate, the impact (steps, calories, and active minutes), or a photo.

7. **Select Share.**

   Fitbit adds the achievement to the Compose screen.

8. **Select Next.**

   Fitbit displays the Share to Community screen, where you should see the Friends option selected in the Closed Groups section. If not, go ahead and select the Friends option.

9. **Select Post.**

   Fitbit posts the message to your friends.

Setting Up a Family Account

If you want to get your kids doing the Fitbit thing, you probably want to get them a Fitbit Ace, which is a tracker designed for kids. (See Chapter 2 for more info on the Ace.) However, to set up the Ace, you first need to create a family account, which is a special subset of your Fitbit friends that has only family members.

Creating a family account

Run through the following steps to get a family account set up in the Fitbit app:

1. **Select Dashboard ⇨ Account to open the Account screen.**

2. **Select Create Family Account.**

   The app displays an overview of the family account.

3. **Select Create Family.**

   The app creates a new family for you and sets you up as the main guardian.

Wow, "guardian" sure sounds impressive, but what does it mean? A family *guardian* can add and remove other guardians, invite family members to join, and create accounts for children, which includes setting up a Fitbit Ace. The next few sections describe these tasks.

Adding a family guardian

Before you can invite a friend to be a guardian, that person must make their birthday info available so that Fitbit can make sure the person is at least 18 years old. So your first chore is to ask all the people who you want to invite to be guardians to make their birthday available to their Fitbit friends. Here are the steps each person needs to follow:

1. **In the Fitbit app, select Dashboard ⇨ Account.**

2. **Select Privacy.**

3. **Select Birthday.**

4. **Select the Friends radio button.**

    Fitbit now makes the person's birthday info visible to friends only.

Friends can also make their birthday info visible using Fitbit.com. They should log in and select View Profile ⇨ View Account Settings ⇨ Privacy (or surf directly to www.fitbit.com/settings/privacy). Next, select Birthday and then select Friends Only.

With that out of the way, to invite one of your Fitbit friends to be a family guardian (which also adds that person to your family account), follow these steps in the Fitbit app:

1. **Select Dashboard ⇨ Account.**

    You need to use the Fitbit app here because there's no way to invite a friend to be a guardian online by using Fitbit.com.

REMEMBER

2. **Select My Family.**

    The app displays the My Family screen.

3. **Select Add Guardians.**

    In the Android app, first tap the Add icon (+) and then tap Add Guardians.

4. **Select the Invite icon beside the person you want to invite to be a guardian.**

    The app sends the invitation to the friend.

Inviting others to the family account

Want to invite an adult family member to join your family account, but you don't want the person to be a guardian? Follow these steps to invite that person:

REMEMBER

1. **Select Dashboard ➪ Account.**

    You need to use the Fitbit app because there's no way to invite people to join your family account online by using Fitbit.com.

2. **Select My Family.**

    The app displays the My Family screen.

3. **Select Invite Members.**

    In the Android app, first tap the Add icon (+) and then tap Invite Members.

4. **Select the Invite icon beside the person you want to invite to join your family account.**

    The app sends the invitation to the friend.

Handling a family invitation

When a family invitation request comes in through Fitbit, one of the following occurs:

>> **Android or Windows 10:** You see a notification onscreen similar to the one shown earlier in Figure 4-3, left. Select View to open the invitation.

>> **iOS:** You see a badge on the Fitbit app's Notifications icon. Tap Notifications, tap Messages if it isn't already displayed, and then tap the invitation.

With the invitation displayed, select Join Family.

Creating a child account

Creating a child account means both setting up an account on Fitbit and pairing an Ace tracker with the Android, iOS, or Windows 10 device the child will use to run a scaled-down version of the Fitbit app. Here's how it works:

1. **On the device your child will use to run the Fitbit app, install the Fitbit app (see Chapter 3), and then use the app to log in to your Fitbit account.**

REMEMBER

2. **Select Dashboard ➪ Account.**

You need to use the Fitbit app because you can't create a child account online by using Fitbit.com.

3. **Select My Family.**

The app displays the My Family screen.

4. **Select Create Child Account.**

In the Android app, first tap the Add icon (+) and then tap Create Child Account.

The app prompts you for your Fitbit account password.

5. **Enter your Fitbit password, and then select Confirm.**

The Fitbit app displays some privacy info.

6. **Select Next, and then select I Agree.**

The Add Child screen appears. The iOS version is shown in Figure 4-10.

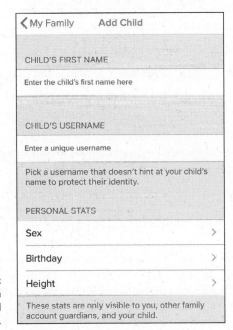

FIGURE 4-10:
The iOS version of the Add Child screen.

REMEMBER

7. **Fill in the child's info, and the select Next.**

If you have an eyebrow raised because Fitbit want to know your child's gender, birthday, and height, know that this information is visible only to you, to any other guardian in your family account, and to the child.

Fitbit prompts you to pair the device with your child's Ace. Make sure the Ace is nearby (within about 33 feet) before proceeding.

8. **Select Pair with This Device. When Fitbit asks you to confirm, select Yes.**

The Fitbit app switches to Kid View, which is the scaled-down app interface that your child will use.

9. **Select Set Up a Kid-Compatible Tracker, and then select Ace.**

10. **Select Set Up Ace for *Name*, where *Name* is your child's name.**

Fitbit displays its terms and policies legal stuff.

11. **Read (wink, wink) the terms and policies, and then select I Agree.**

Fitbit displays several introductory screens for the Ace tracker.

12. **Select Next on each screen until the Fitbit app locates the Ace tracker.**

Fitbit displays a four-digit number on the Ace display.

13. **In the Fitbit app, enter the four-digit number to pair the device to the Ace.**

If you see a screen telling you that an update is available for the tracker, select Update Ace.

14. **Follow the onscreen introduction to the Ace tracker by selecting Next on each screen that appears.**

When the introduction is complete, the app displays the Dashboard in Kid View.

REMEMBER

On your child's device, if you want full access to all Fitbit app features and settings, you need to switch to Parent View. Select Dashboard ➪ Account ➪ Switch to Parent View. When the app asks you to confirm, select Switch to Parent View, enter your Fitbit password, and then select Confirm. To return to Kid View, select Dashboard ➪ Account ➪ My Family, select the child's account in the Children section, and then select Switch to Kid View.

TIP

If you need to delete a child account, select Dashboard ➪ Account ➪ My Family to display your family members. In the Android app, tap and hold down on the child's name, and then tap Remove; in the iOS app, swipe left on the child's name, and then tap Remove; in the Windows 10 app, tap the Edit icon (pencil) and then select the Remove icon (X) next to the child's account. In all versions of the app, you now select Delete Child Account & Data, enter your Fitbit password, and then select Confirm.

Joining In the Group Fun

Interacting with friends and family on Fitbit is fun and motivating, but it doesn't represent all of Fitbit's social side. A large collection of *groups*, which are collections of like-minded Fitbit users, is available. Each group is devoted to a particular theme — such as Walking, Running, Heart Health, and Strength Training (to name four popular groups) — and anyone who joins a group can post their Fitbit achievements and workouts and view the posts of other group members.

Joining an existing group

Fitbit offers a curated list of groups in the Fitbit app. Here's how to join one of those groups:

1. **Select Community.**

2. **Select the Groups tab.**

3. **Select Discover More Groups.**

   The app displays a few groups, organized into categories such as Eat Well and Get Moving.

4. **If you see a group you like, select it to open the group, view a description, and peruse some recent posts.**

5. **If you like what you see, select Join.**

   Fitbit adds you to the group.

Viewing group posts

To see the latest goings-on in a group you've joined, follow these steps:

1. **Select Community.**

2. **Select the Groups tab.**

3. **Select the group you want to view.**

   Fitbit displays the group screen and shows the posts in reverse chronological order (that is, the most recent posts appear at the top).

TIP

If you end up joining multiple groups, you might not feel like visiting each group separately to catch up. Instead, select the Community tab and then select the Feed tab, which displays the most recent posts from all your groups.

TECHNICAL STUFF

CREATING YOUR OWN GROUP

When you display the Fitbit app's Community section and select the Groups tab, you see a curated list of groups that you can join. However, the Groups tab also includes an intriguing command at the top: Create a Group. Yep, that's right: Fitbit enables you to build a group with your bare hands. Your group won't appear in the Groups tab, but it does appear in the Groups page of Fitbit.com, which you can eyeball for yourself by surfing to www.fitbit.com and selecting Community ⇨ Activity Group, or by heading directly to www.fitbit.com/groups.

The Groups page contains thousands of groups. Most have just single-digit memberships, but some have hundreds of even thousands of members. To join one of these groups, select it and then select Join This Group. If you can't access the group, it means the group is private, and therefore not open to the likes of you and me, or is invitation-only.

If you have a great idea for a group, or if you want to create a group for your sports team, running club, workplace, school, or just some random collection of acquaintances, follow these steps in the Fitbit app:

1. **Select Community ⇨ Groups.**

2. **Select Create a Group.**

3. **Select Get Started.**

4. **Select the camera icon that appears beside the default header image, and then add a header image for the group.**

   You can use your device's camera or upload a photo).

5. **In the Group Name text box, enter a name for your group (25 characters max).**

6. **In the Description text box to enter a description for your group (100 characters max).**

7. **In the Group Rules text box, enter a rundown of your group's rules (5,000 characters max)**

8. **Select Create (Android or iOS) or Next (Windows 10).**

   Fitbit prompts you to invite some friends to the group.

9. **Select Invite, select the radio button beside each friend you want to invite, and then select Send.**

If you want to create a private or invitation-only group, you need to use Fitbit.com and the following steps:

1. Go to www.fitbit.com and log in to your account.

2. Select Community ⇨ Activity Groups, or go directly to www.fitbit.com/groups.

3. Select Create a Group.

4. Enter a group name and a group description.

5. If you want group members to join only if they get an invitation, select the Public, Invitation Only option.

6. If you want the group to be hidden to others, select the Private option.

7. Select Create.

   Fitbit.com creates the group.

Responding to group posts

When you're viewing a group's posts, you might get the overwhelming urge to respond to a post. No problem. Fitbit offers two ways to respond by adding the following two icons below every post:

>> **Cheer:** Send a cheer to the person who posted the message.

>> **Comment:** Send the person a message, which appears below the post when you select the post in your feed.

Posting a message to a group

It's fine to be a group *lurker* — that is, someone who just reads other people's posts — when you first join a group. However, after you have a feel for the group, why not post an impressive Dashboard, a workout you're proud of, or just your couple of cents' worth? When you're ready to share, follow these steps:

1. Select Community.

2. Select the Groups tab.

3. **Select the group to which you want to post.**

Fitbit displays the group's home screen, which includes a What Are You Up To? text box near the top, as shown in Figure 4-11.

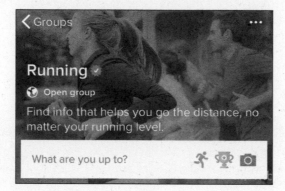

FIGURE 4-11:
Each group home page includes a text box.

4. **Select the What Are You Up To? text box.**

Fitbit open the Compose screen, which includes both a text box for a message and several buttons for sharing achievements, as shown in Figure 4-12.

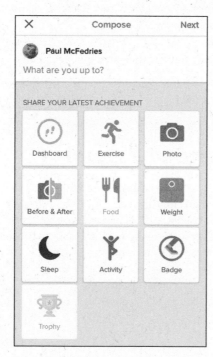

FIGURE 4-12:
The Compose screen includes a text box and buttons for sharing achievements.

5. **In the What Are You Up To? text box, type a message.**

6. **To share an achievement:**

   a. *Tap the corresponding button, and then use the screen that appears to select the specific achievement you want to share.*

   b. *If the achievement has display options, select the options you want to use.* For example, with a walk or run you can display the exercise heart rate, impact (steps, calories, and active minutes), or a photo.

   c. *Select Share.*

   Fitbit adds the achievement to the Compose screen.

7. **Select Next.**

   Fitbit displays the Share to Community screen, where you should see your group selected in the Open Groups section. If not, go ahead and select your group.

8. **Select Post.**

   Fitbit posts the message to the group.

2

Tracking Your Health and Fitness

IN THIS CHAPTER

» Setting your activity goals

» Tracking steps and active minutes

» Setting hourly reminders to move

» Tracking distance floors climbed

» Earning badges to commemorate your hard work

Chapter 5

Tracking Your Daily Activity Levels

"Use it or lose it." "No pain no gain." "The hardest part is walking out the front door." "The only bad workout is no workout."

"Turn fat into fit." "It never gets easier. You just get strong." "Pain is just weakness leaving your body."

The fitness world has never found a cliché or bromide that it wouldn't put on a poster and slap on a gym wall.

Ah, but here's the thing: If you could scrub the encrusted triteness and staleness off each of these platitudes, you'd be left with a shining gem of truth. Yep, as hackneyed as these slogans appear, each of them is unarguably, unassailably true. You really do lose mobility and muscle if you don't give your body movement and resistance. Your body really does improve only if you stress it a little. Doing nothing really is worse than doing something.

In this chapter, you bring these slogans off the gym wall and into your life. In the pages that follow, you explore all the Fitbit features and settings related to tracking your daily activities, including steps, hourly activity, active minutes, distance, and floors climbed.

"Just do it."

Setting Activity Goals

Undertaking an exercise program without setting a goal is like taking the family on a driving trip without choosing a destination. Sure, it will probably be fun at the beginning, but eventually it will devolve into aimless wandering and sullen silence. Your health is too important to let that happen, so you need to define goals for the Fitbit metrics you want to track.

REMEMBER

If you're not sure what goal to set for yourself, skip this step for now and use your Fitbit for a few days to see what stats you generate. If you find that, say, you're doing 5,000 steps most days, try setting your daily step goal at 6,000 to challenge yourself a bit.

Setting your daily activity goals

Here are the steps to follow to set your daily activity goals:

1. **In the Fitbit app, click Dashboard ⇨ Account.**

   The Account screen appears.

2. **In the Goals section, click the Activity tab.**

   Fitbit displays the Activity Goals screen. Figure 5-1 shows the iOS version of the screen.

‹ Account Activity Goals	
Daily Activity	
Steps	10,000 steps
Distance	6 km
Calories Burned	2,000 cals
Active Minutes	40 minutes
Floors Climbed	10 floors
Hourly Activity Goal	11 hr/day

FIGURE 5-1:
The iOS version of the Activity Goals screen.

3. **Click Steps and then type the number of steps you want to shoot for each day.**

4. **Click Distance and then enter the daily distance you want to reach.**

5. **Click Calories Burned and then type the number of calories you want to expend each day.**

6. **Click Active Minutes and then type the number of minutes you'd like to be active daily.**

7. **Click Floors Climbed and then type the number of floors you hope to ascend each day.**

   Wait: What about hourly activity? Yup, I cover that; see the section "Staying Regular: Setting Hourly Activity Goals and Reminders," later in this chapter.

8. **Click the Back icon (<) to return to the Account screen.**

   The Fitbit app syncs the new goals to your Fitbit device.

Setting your main activity goal

In Fitbit land, your *main goal* is the metric that Fitbit tracks most closely, which means two things:

>> In the Fitbit app's Today section, Fitbit.com's Today tile, and the Today app on the Ionic or Versa watch, the main goal is the metric you see first.

>> When you reach your main goal, your Fitbit vibrates in a celebratory way and displays a notification congratulating you on reaching your goal.

The steps metric is the default main goal, but you can follow this procedure to specify a different main goal:

1. **In the Fitbit app, click Dashboard ⇨ Account.**

   The Account screen appears.

2. **Click your Fitbit device.**

3. **Click Main Goal.**

   The Main Goal screen appears.

4. **Click the activity you want to use as your main goal.**

5. **Click the Back icon (<) until you return to the Account screen.**

   The Fitbit app syncs the new main goal to your Fitbit device.

Left, Right, Left, Right: Counting Your Steps

The simplest and most basic activity you can do is to put one foot in front of the other, and then repeat as often as possible or as necessary. The humble step might seem *too* humble to serve as an engine of health or fitness, but make no mistake: Walking is fantastic exercise that has both physical and mental benefits. Yes, generally speaking, the faster you take those steps, the greater the benefits, but even a modest stroll or amble is *way* better than plopping yourself, potato-like, on your couch.

The idea that walking at any speed is superior to sitting at no speed is inherent in the default stat monitored by all Fitbit trackers: the step. To your Fitbit, a step is a step, whether it's taken during a leisurely saunter or a full-on sprint. What your Fitbit really cares about is the *number* of steps you take each day, not the speed at which you take them. That makes sense because the more steps you take, the more time you're active during the day, so the *less* time you're sitting around. (That said, your Fitbit *does* differentiate between slow and fast activities; see "Earning Active Minutes," later in this chapter.)

Monitoring today's steps

You'll want to keep an eye peeled on your step count throughout the day to make sure you reach your goal. Fortunately, Fitbit gives you many ways to do this:

REMEMBER

>> **Ace, Alta, or Alta HR:** Wake the Fitbit and then tap the screen until you see the step count.

   On most of the Fitbit platforms, the steps metric is indicated by the two footprints icon, which is labeled in Figure 5-2, left.

>> **Charge 3, Inspire, or Inspire HR:** Wake the device and then swipe up.

>> **Flex 2:** Four of the five LEDs indicate your progress. One LED lights up when you hit 25 percent of your goal; a second LED lights when you hit 50 percent; a third LED lights when you get to 75 percent, and all four LEDs are lit and the fifth LED turns green when you reach your goal.

>> **Ionic or Versa:** You have two choices:

   ● Wake the device, display the clock (if it's not displayed already), and then tap the screen. Figure 5-2, left, shows the step count as it appears on the Ionic watch. Note, too, the steps goal circle in the upper-right corner, which shows you how much of your daily steps goal you've achieved so far.

   ● Wake the device, display the clock (if it's not displayed already), and then swipe up from the bottom of the screen to open the Today app, which initially shows the step count and the steps goal circle, as shown in Figure 5-2, right. (If you see some other metric, then steps isn't defined as your main goal; see "Setting your main activity goal," earlier in this chapter.)

» **Fitbit app:** Open the Dashboard. Today's step count appears near the top of the screen, as shown in Figure 5-3.

» **Fitbit.com:** Log in to your Fitbit account to open the Dashboard. Today's step count appears in the Today tile. To see what percentage of your steps goal you've achieved, hover the mouse pointer over the Today tile, as shown in Figure 5-4.

How much of your daily goal you've achieved

Steps metric

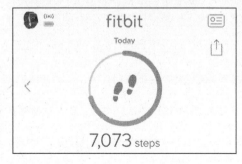

FIGURE 5-2: See the current step count by tapping the watch clock (left) or opening the Today app.

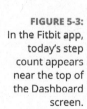

FIGURE 5-3: In the Fitbit app, today's step count appears near the top of the Dashboard screen.

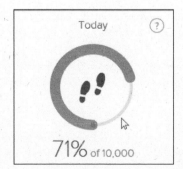

FIGURE 5-4: In the Fitbit.com Dashboard, hover the mouse over the Today tile to change the counts to percentages.

DO YOU REALLY NEED TO DO 10,000 STEPS?

Just before the 1964 Summer Olympics in Tokyo, a Japanese company came out with an early version of a pedometer which they described as a *manpo-kei,* the literal translation of which is "10,000 steps meter." The hook, you see, was to get Japanese walkers to go from the 1,000 to 3,000 steps each person might take during a typical day to 10,000 daily steps to improve fitness and lose weight. That 10,000 number was based on hard science, right? Not even close. It was dreamt up by the marketing department because 10,000 is an auspicious number in Japanese culture. That auspiciousness was probably why the number was embraced by the Japanese public, and the popularity in Japan was probably why word soon spread around the world that everybody should aim for 10,000 steps every day.

10,000 *is* an awfully nice number, so why not make it everyone's goal? The problem is that 10,000 steps is trying to be a one-size-fits-all solution in a world where size variations are too numerous and too varied. Think about it: Doesn't it seem a little far-fetched that a single number should apply to every person on the planet? Whether you're large or small, young or old, fit or fat, athlete or couch potato, you *must* walk 10,000 steps! It doesn't make sense, and many scientific studies have concluded that 10,000 steps doesn't work for every person.

So when you're setting your daily steps goal, don't just plug in 10,000 and move on. If you're starting out, perhaps 5,000 steps is a good goal for you. If you have a dog that you take on a couple of walks a day, perhaps 15,000 steps is a more realistic goal. You should come up with a number that suits — and challenges — you and your lifestyle, not what some 1960s Japanese marketing team came up with.

Viewing your steps history

Although it's important to regularly check your progress towards your daily steps goal, it's just as important to occasionally glance back at your past step counts. In this way, you can detect patterns, see when it's time to increase your daily steps goal, and set appropriate challenges.

Assuming you've synced your Fitbit device recently, you can view your steps history by using the Dashboard on either the Fitbit app or the Fitbit.com website:

> » In the Dashboard, click the Previous icon (<) to go back one day (see Figure 5-5). After you've gone back one or more days, you can click the Next icon (>) to move forward a day.

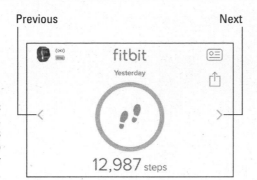

Previous   Next

FIGURE 5-5:
In the Dashboard,
click the Previous
and Next icons to
navigate your
steps history.

>> In the Dashboard, click the steps metric. Fitbit opens the Steps screen,
which displays a chart of the previous seven days' step counts and how
they compare to your steps goal, as shown in Figure 5-6. You can also scroll
down to see the step counts from previous days, and you can click any day
to see a timeline of when the steps occurred during the day, as shown in
Figure 5-7.

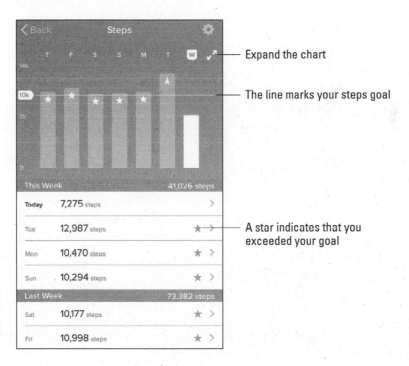

Expand the chart

The line marks your steps goal

A star indicates that you
exceeded your goal

FIGURE 5-6:
The Steps
screen displays
your historical
steps data.

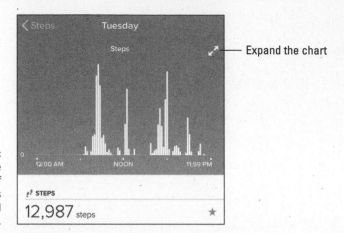

— Expand the chart

FIGURE 5-7:
Click a day to see
a timeline of
when your steps
occurred
that day.

Staying Regular: Setting Hourly Activity Goals and Reminders

Being active during the day involves two components:

>> The total activity you perform during the day

>> The activity you perform regularly throughout the day

It's important to separate these two components of activity because each is crucial to your health. For example, suppose you set a goal of 8,000 steps each day and you then go out on a single long walk that gets you over the 8,000-step hump. Nice work! However, if you then sit around for the rest of the day, all that sitting *negates* the benefits of your walk! It's unfair, I know, but sitting really is that bad for you.

So what's the solution? You need to move *throughout* the day, not just in a single burst. Fortunately, Fitbit's got your back on this one because you can set up your tracker to give you hourly nudges to get up and move. It works like this: Fitbit tracks the number of steps you take each hour. If your step count is less than 250 as the end of the hour approaches (specifically, at ten minutes to the hour), your Fitbit vibrates and displays a reminder, similar to the one shown in Figure 5-8.

REMEMBER

If you have a Fitbit Flex 2, your reminder to move is a vibration accompanied by a single purple light and two white lights.

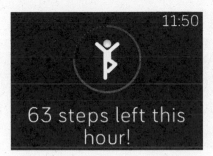

FIGURE 5-8:
If you haven't reached 250 steps this hour, Fitbit tells you to get a move on.

250 steps is just two or three minutes walking for most people, so why not take a short break and move around a bit? As a reward, if you hit 250 steps before the hour is up, your Fitbit offers a brief celebratory message, as shown in Figure 5-9).

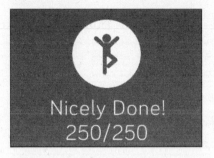

FIGURE 5-9:
Your Fitbit celebrates if you reach 250 steps before the hour ends.

Checking your hourly steps

If you don't want to wait until ten minutes to the hour to check your hourly steps, you can monitor your progress if you have one of the following Fitbit devices:

» **Charge 3, Inspire, or Inspire HR:** Wake the device, and then swipe up until you see a person walking icon with the caption *x* of 250, where *x* is the number of steps you've taken so far this hour.

» **Ionic or Versa:** Wake the device, display the clock, and swipe up from the bottom of the screen to launch the Today app. Then swipe up until you see a screen similar to the one in Figure 5-10 with the text *x* Steps This Hour, where *x* is the number of steps you've taken so far this hour.

REMEMBER

If you don't see your hourly steps on your Fitbit device, it means you've already met your goal for this hour. Good work!

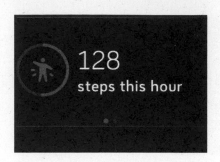

Setting up hourly reminders to move

Your Fitbit's hourly prods to get up and move are one of its best features because — let's face it — most of us need prodding! Even better is the fact that you can customize which hours during the day your hourly steps goal is in effect.

Here are the steps to follow using either the Fitbit app or Fitbit.com to configure your hourly reminders to move:

1. **Click Dashboard ⇨ Account.**

   The Accounts screen appears.

2. **Click your Fitbit device.**

3. **Click Reminders to Move.**

   The Reminders to Move screen appears. Figure 5-11 shows the iOS version of the screen.

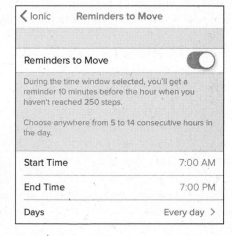

4. **If you want to receive reminders each hour, make sure the Reminders to Move switch is on (green).**

5. **Use the Start Time list to specify the first hour you want Fitbit to track your hourly steps. Use the End Time list to specify the last hour you want Fitbit to track your hourly steps.**

   In the Android app, tap Start & End Time, enter the start and end hour, and then tap OK.

   Each hour from the start time until the end time, Fitbit will check whether you've taken at least 250 steps. If you haven't reached 250 by ten minutes before the hour is done, your Fitbit will vibrate and display a reminder.

6. **If you are using the Fitbit app, click Days.**

7. **Select which days of the week you want Fitbit to track your hourly steps.**

8. **If you're using Fitbit.com, click Save.**

   Fitbit saves your settings.

Monitoring today's hourly activity

When you're just starting out with your fitness program, it's easy to forget to move each hour, mostly because not moving is such a habit for most of us. So at first your hourly activity will only be "hourly-ish." To improve, you need to monitor this metric and let the gaps in your activity motivate you to do better tomorrow.

Here are the various ways that Fitbit offers to monitor today's hourly activity:

>> **Ace, Alta, Alta HR, or Flex 2:** These devices don't show hourly activity, so you need to use the Fitbit app or Fitbit.com, as I describe later in this list.

>> **Charge 3, Inspire, or Inspire HR:** Wake the device and then swipe up until you see the *x* of *y* value (where *x* is the number of hours you've met your goal and *y* is the total number of hours you're tracking).

>> **Ionic or Versa:** Wake the device, display the clock (if it's not displayed already), and then swipe up from the bottom of the screen to open the Today app. Swipe up until you see the *x* of *y* Hours Today value (where *x* is the number of hours you've met your goal and *y* is the total number of hours you're tracking), as shown in Figure 5-12, left. If, instead, you see *x* Steps This Hour, swipe left on it.

REMEMBER

On most Fitbit platforms, the hourly activity metric is indicated by an icon showing a person with arms raised and one foot braced against the other leg (the Tree pose in yoga), as labeled in Figure 5-12, right.

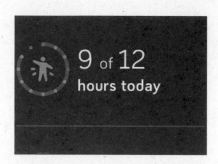
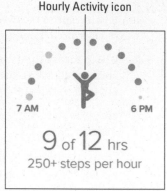

Hourly Activity icon

7 AM   6 PM

9 of 12 hrs
250+ steps per hour

FIGURE 5-12:
The hourly activity metric in the Today app (left) and in the Fitbit app's Dashboard (right).

>> **Fitbit app:** Open the Dashboard and view the *x* of *y* Hrs value, as shown in Figure 5-12, right.

>> **Fitbit.com:** Log in to your Fitbit account to open the Dashboard, and then view the *x* of *y* Hrs tile.

Viewing your hourly activity history

After you've tracked your hourly activity for a while, a question might arise: Are there particular hours when I'm regularly inactive? For example, perhaps you always miss your 250-step goal between 4 p.m. and 5 p.m. (presumably because you hunker down at your desk to complete some work before leaving at 5).

You could figure this out by using the Dashboard on the Fitbit app or on Fitbit.com to navigate through the previous days, looking for patterns. However, a much easier way is to open the Dashboard and then click the hourly activity metric. Fitbit opens the Hourly Activity screen shown in Figure 5-13, which displays a chart of the previous seven days, broken down by hour, with a dot placed on each hour you met your 250-step goal. This display gives you a quick way to see persistent gaps in your activity.

Viewing your stationary time

It's hard to get through the day without seeing a headline of the form "Sitting is the new *x*," where *x* is smoking or sugar or cancer or some other very bad thing. I talk about this in greater detail in Chapter 11, but for now let me just say that about a billion studies have proven that sitting too much is extremely bad for you. Therefore, although being active throughout the day is vital to your overall health, it's also important to keep an eye on how much time you *don't* move during the day. You should be aware of two stats when you monitor your stationary time:

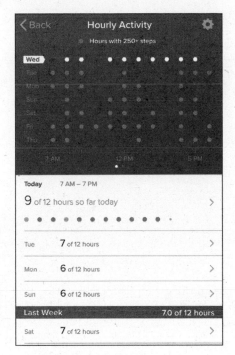

FIGURE 5-13:
The Hourly Activity screen breaks down the last week by hour.

>> The longest stationary period during the day

>> The total amount of time you're stationary during the day — expressed as the number of hours and minutes you don't move or as a percentage of the total time

To monitor these stats, follow these steps:

1. **Open the Dashboard on either the Fitbit app or Fitbit.com.**

2. **Click the hourly activity metric.**

    The Hourly Activity screen appears.

3. **Click the day you want to examine.**

    Fitbit displays a summary of that day's hourly activity, as shown in Figure 5-14. The summary includes values for Longest Stationary Period and All Day Breakdown, which displays the stationary time as a total and as a percentage.

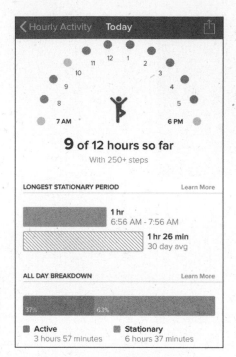

FIGURE 5-14:
The hourly activity summary includes stats for longest and total stationary time.

Earning Active Minutes

Earlier in this chapter I mentioned that any activity is good for heart and mind because moving is always better than sitting down or standing in one place. I stand by (walk with?) that, but it doesn't tell the entire story. Yes, it's true that moving is good, but moving moderately faster is better than moving slowly. When you pick up the pace to a brisk walk, a determined march, or even a slow jog, your heart rate goes up, your muscles work a bit harder, and you burn more calories.

Whatever your goal — getting fit, losing some fat, or dropping a few pounds — you won't get there unless some of your activity can be characterized as moderately intense. Fitbit describes time spent in moderate intensity (or faster) activities as *active minutes*, and in this section I tell you all you need to know about this crucial metric.

Understanding metabolic equivalents

Okay, so let me start with the question that I'm sure you're shouting at the book right now, "How do I define *moderately intense*?" One straightforward way is to compare the energy (calories) you use during an activity with the energy you use when you're not doing anything. A body at rest still expends some energy to keep the lights on, so to speak (that is, keep the heart beating, the lungs breathing, food digesting, and so on). The rate of energy you expend is called your *metabolic rate*.

To compare different types of activities, exercise eggheads came up with a measure called metabolic equivalent of task, or MET. One *MET* is defined as the amount of energy you expend when you're at rest. If you do something that expends twice as much energy as you do at rest, that activity is said to require two METs of energy expenditure.

Okay, we're almost there. We can now use METs to define three types of activity intensity based on how much energy they require you to expend:

>> **Easy intensity:** Any activity that requires less than three METs. For example, walking at two miles per hour (very slow indeed) expends 2.5 METs. On an effort scale of 0 to 10 (where 0 is doing nothing and 10 is as hard as you can go), easy activities feel like a 3 or a 4. Your breathing and heart rate should stay normal or show at most a slight increase.

>> **Moderate intensity:** Any activity that requires at least three METs but less than six METs. For example, walking at three miles per hour (a decent pace) expends 3.5 METs, while kicking it up to four miles per hour (very brisk) expends 5 METs. On an effort scale of 0 to 10, moderate activities feel like a 5 or a 6. Your breathing and heart rate should show a noticeable increase.

>> **Vigorous intensity:** Any activity that requires at least six METs. For example, jogging at six miles per hour (ten minutes per mile) expends 9.8 METs. On an effort scale of 0 to 10, vigorous activities feel like a 7 or an 8. Your breathing and heart rate should show large increases, but you shouldn't feel completely out of breath.

Okay, so you go out and walk at three or four miles per hour for 60 seconds and you earn yourself an active minute on your Fitbit Dashboard, right? Not so fast, friend. For a moderate intensity (or vigorous intensity) activity to do you good, it must be maintained for at least ten minutes. Therefore, you get credit for active minutes on your Fitbit only if you perform a moderate or vigorous intensity activity for at least ten minutes.

Table 5-1 shows a few activities and the METs they expend.

TABLE 5-1 **Example Activities and Their METs**

Activity	METs
Easy intensity (< 3.0)	
Light household cleaning (dusting, sweeping, and so on)	2.3
Walking at 2.0 mph	2.5
Walking at 2.5 mph	2.9
Moderate intensity (>= 3.0 and < 6.0)	
Walking at 3.0 mph	3.5
Moderate outdoor work (digging, spading, and so on)	3.5
Moderate household cleaning (vacuuming, mopping, cleaning windows, and so on)	3.5
Moderate outdoor work (raking leaves, trimming shrubs, weeding, and so on)	4.0
Pushing a stroller at 3.0 mph	4.0
Climbing stairs (slow)	4.0
Golf (no cart; carrying your clubs)	4.3
Chopping wood (moderate effort)	4.5
Walking at 4.0 mph	5.0
Kayaking (moderate effort)	5.0
Skiing or snowboarding (moderate effort)	5.3
Canoeing (moderate effort)	5.8
Swimming (moderate effort)	5.8
Vigorous intensity (>= 6.0)	
Vigorous outdoor work (hand mowing, shoveling snow, and so on)	6.3
Dancing	7.8
Hiking with a daypack	7.8
Walking at 3.0 mph uphill (6% to 15% grade)	8.0
Climbing stairs (fast)	8.8
Swimming (vigorous effort)	9.8
Running at 6 mph (10 minutes per mile)	9.8
Running at 6.7 mph (9 minutes per mile)	10.5
Running at 7.5 mph (8 minutes per mile)	11.8
Running up stairs	15

Monitoring today's active minutes

Most health and fitness professionals recommend that children, adults, and seniors should perform a minimum number of minutes of moderate intensity activity per week. The specific minimums vary, but the following are the most common:

» **Children (ages 6 and up):** At least 60 minutes per day

» **Adults:** At least 150 minutes per week (about 22 minutes per day)

» **Seniors:** At least 150 minutes per week, or as many minutes as health and physical ability will allow

Use these numbers to set your daily goal for the active minutes metric (see "Setting your daily activity goals," earlier in the chapter), and then use Fitbit to monitor your active minutes throughout the day:

REMEMBER

» **Ace, Alta, or Alta HR:** Wake the Fitbit and then tap the screen until you see the active minutes.

On most Fitbit platforms, the active minutes metric is indicated by the lightning bolt icon.

» **Charge 3, Inspire, or Inspire HR:** Wake the device and then swipe up until you see the active minutes.

» **Flex 2:** This device doesn't show active minutes, so you need to use either the Fitbit app or Fitbit.com, as I describe later in this list.

» **Ionic or Versa:** Wake the device, display the clock (if it's not displayed already), and then swipe up from the bottom of the screen to open the Today app, which initially shows today's step count. Swipe left until you see the active minutes value, shown in Figure 5-15, left.

» **Fitbit app:** Open the Dashboard and view the active minutes metric, pointed out in Figure 5-15, right.

» **Fitbit.com:** Log in to your Fitbit account to open the Dashboard, and then view the Active Minutes tile.

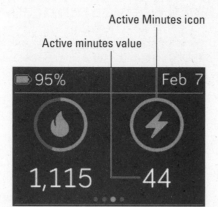
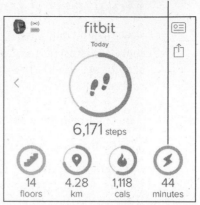

FIGURE 5-15: Active minutes in the Today app (left) and as it appears in the Fitbit app's Dashboard (right).

Active minutes value

Active Minutes icon

Active minutes

Viewing your active minutes history

If you want to get a larger sense of how you're doing with the active minutes metric, you need to go beyond what's happening today and dive into your historical data. By studying the active minutes you've accumulated on previous days, you can see how often you're meeting your goal and whether you need to adjust that goal up or down.

Assuming you've synced your Fitbit device recently, you can view your active minutes history by using the Dashboard on either the Fitbit app or the Fitbit.com website:

>> In the Dashboard, click the Previous icon (<) to go back one day. After you've gone back one or more days, you can also click the Next icon (>) to move forward a day.

>> In the Dashboard, click the active minutes metric. Fitbit opens the Active Minutes screen, which displays a chart of the previous seven days' worth of active minutes and how they compare to your goal, as shown in Figure 5-16. You can scroll down to see the active minutes from previous days, and you can click any day to see a timeline of when the active minutes occurred.

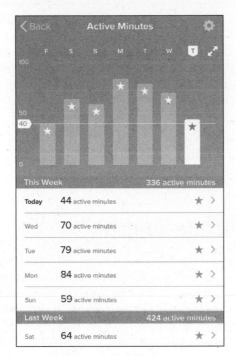

FIGURE 5-16:
The Active
Minutes screen
displays your
historical active
minutes data.

Going the Distance: Measuring How Far You Walked or Ran

Unless you're a runner or a cyclist, the distance you cover during the day is less important than either the number of steps you take or the active minutes you chalk up. However, that doesn't mean that you should ignore Fitbit's distance metric, because it can be a good indicator of improving fitness. For example, suppose when you were starting out you walked for 30 minutes and your Fitbit said that you covered 1.5 miles during that walk. Now, six months later, for that same 30-minute walk, your Fitbit says that you covered 2 miles. That 33 percent distance increase means you're walking faster, which tells you you're getting fitter.

How does your Fitbit know how far you've propelled yourself during the day? It depends:

>> All Fitbit devices that track distance do so by multiplying the number of steps you take by the length of your stride. That stride length is an educated guess on Fitbit's part based on your height and gender. Note, too, that Fitbit stores *two* stride lengths for you: one for walking and another for running

>> The Fitbit Ionic watch comes with its own GPS (Global Positioning System) receiver, so it uses that signal to track your location and calculate the distance you travel. Note that the device uses GPS for only certain activities that you initiate using the Exercise app, such as running and walking. (See Chapter 9 for details.) The Ionic doesn't use GPS for regularly tracked activities.

>> The Fitbit Versa watch and the Charge 3 and Inspire HR wristbands piggyback on your smartphone's GPS receiver and calculate your distance using that signal. As with the Ionic, these trackers use GPS only for activities initiated through the Exercise app.

Setting your stride length

Given the height and gender info that you gave when setting up your Fitbit account (see Chapter 3), Fitbit uses some standard calculations to come up with lengths for your walking and running strides. Those calculations usually work fine for most people, but some of us have legs that are shorter or longer than average, while others have walking or running mechanics that dictate a stride length that's shorter or longer than average. Any of these anomalies could cause the distance calculation to be too short or too long. Fortunately, if that's the case for you, Fitbit enables you to edit your calculated stride lengths with your actual stride values.

TIP

If you have a Fitbit that uses GPS, each time you go on a run of at least ten minutes, the device compares the distance you ran (determined via GPS) to the distance the device thinks you ran (calculated by multiplying your steps by your running stride length). If there's a discrepancy, Fitbit adjusts your running stride length measure so that the distance calculation matches the GPS value.

How do you figure out the lengths of your walking and running strides? Here's the easiest method:

1. Find a running track or some other route or trail where you know the exact distance.

2. Walk at you're your normal pace one lap around the track (or whatever) and count your strides (both left and right) as you go.

3. Divide the distance you walked — in feet or centimeters, depending on which measurement you're using — by the total number of strides you took to traverse the distance. For example, if the lap is 440 yards (5,280 feet) and you took 1,800 strides, your stride length is 5,280 ÷ 1,800, or 2.9 feet.

4. Repeat Steps 1 through 3 for your running stride, but run instead of walk in Step 2.

You're now ready to enter your custom stride lengths in your Fitbit account.

Entering custom stride lengths by using the Fitbit app

Follow these steps to use the Fitbit app to plug in your custom stride lengths:

1. **Click Dashboard ⇨ Account.**

2. **Click Advanced Settings.**

3. **Click Stride Length.**

   The Stride Length screen appears.

4. **Click the Set Automatically switch to off.**

   In the Windows 10 app, click the Auto switch to off.

5. **In the Walking Stride Length box, enter the length of your walking stride.**

6. **In the Running Stride Length box, enter the length of your running stride.**

7. **Click the Back icon (<) until you reach the Account screen, click your device, and then click Sync.**

   Your Fitbit device now uses your custom stride lengths for its distance calculations.

Entering custom stride lengths by using Fitbit.com

Follow these steps to use Fitbit.com to specify your custom stride lengths:

1. **Surf to www.fitbit.com and log in to display the Dashboard.**

2. **Click View Settings ⇨ Settings.**

3. **Under the Advanced Settings heading, click Stride Length.**

   The Stride Length screen appears.

4. **Select the Set Your Own button.**

5. **In the Walking box, enter your length of your walking stride.**

6. **In the Running box, enter your length of your running stride.**

7. **Click Submit.**

   The next time you sync your Fitbit, the device will use your custom stride lengths for distance calculations.

Monitoring today's distance

Following are the various ways that Fitbit offers to monitor your daily distance:

REMEMBER

» **Ace, Alta, or Alta HR:** Wake the Fitbit and then tap the screen until you see the distance value.

On most Fitbit platforms, the distance metric is indicated by the map marker icon (similar to the location marker in mapping software such as Google Maps), labeled in Figure 5-17, left.

» **Charge 3, Inspire, or Inspire HR:** Wake the device and then swipe up until you see the distance.

» **Flex 2:** This device doesn't show distance, so you need to use either the Fitbit app or Fitbit.com, as I describe later in this list.

» **Ionic or Versa:** Wake the device, display the clock (if it's not displayed already), and then swipe up from the bottom of the screen to open the Today app, which initially shows today's step count. Swipe left until you see the distance metric, shown in Figure 5-17, left.

» **Fitbit app:** Open the Dashboard and view the distance metric, as shown in Figure 5-17, right.

» **Fitbit.com:** Log in to your Fitbit account to open the Dashboard, and then view the Distance tile.

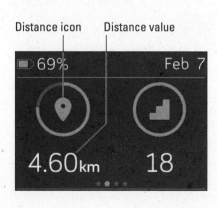
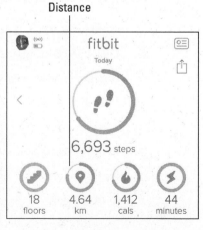

FIGURE 5-17: The distance metric in the Today app (left) and in the Fitbit app's Dashboard (right).

Viewing your active minutes history

If you've set a daily distance goal (see "Setting your daily activity goals," earlier in the chapter), you can monitor how you're doing by eyeballing your distance history using the Dashboard on either the Fitbit app or the Fitbit.com website:

» In the Dashboard, click the Previous icon (<) to go back one day. After you've gone back one or more days, you can also click Next icon (>) to move forward a day.

» In the Dashboard, click the distance metric. Fitbit opens the Distance screen, which displays a chart of the previous seven days of distance values and how they compare to your goal, as shown in Figure 5-18. You can also scroll down to see the distances from previous days, and you can click any day to see a timeline of when the distances occurred during the day.

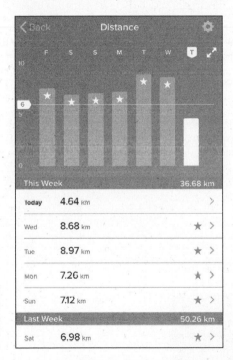

FIGURE 5-18:
The Distance screen displays your historical distance data.

Moving on Up: Tracking Floors Climbed

If you glance back at Table 5-1, you'll see that although slow walking (at two mph) expends a mere 2 METs, climbing the stairs at a slow pace requires double the energy: 4 METs. Climb those same stairs at a quick pace, and your energy output climbs to an impressive 8.8 METs.

Clearly, climbing — whether it's ascending one or more flights of stairs or going up a hill or an inclined road — is great exercise. All the more reason to monitor Fitbit's floors climbed metric, where Fitbit (using its built-in altimeter) defines a *floor* as a climb of ten vertical feet.

Monitoring today's floors climbed

Assuming you've set your daily goal for the floors climbed metric (see "Setting your daily activity goals," earlier in this chapter), here's how to use Fitbit to monitor your floors climbed throughout the day:

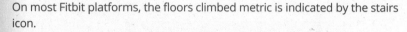

>> **Ace, Alta, or Alta HR:** Wake the Fitbit and then tap the screen until you see the floors climbed.

   On most Fitbit platforms, the floors climbed metric is indicated by the stairs icon.

>> **Charge 3, Inspire, or Inspire HR:** Wake the device and then swipe up until you see the floors climbed.

>> **Flex 2:** This device doesn't show floors climbed, so you need to use either the Fitbit app or Fitbit.com, as I describe later in this list.

>> **Ionic or Versa:** Wake the device, display the clock (if it's not displayed already), and then swipe up from the bottom of the screen to open the Today app, which initially shows today's step count. Swipe left until you see the floors climbed value, shown in Figure 5-19, left.

Floors climbed

Floors climbed value

Floors Climbed icon

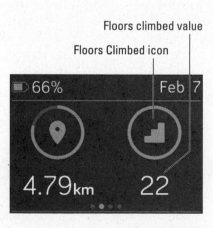

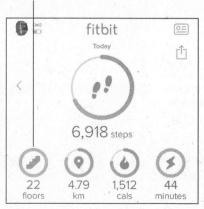

FIGURE 5-19:
The floors climbed metric in the Today app (left) and in the Fitbit app's Dashboard (right).

» **Fitbit app:** Open the Dashboard and view the floors climbed metric, labeled in Figure 5-19, right.

» **Fitbit.com:** Log in to your Fitbit account to open the Dashboard, and then view the floors climbed tile.

Viewing your floors climbed history

To look for patterns in your floors climbed data and to see how you're doing with respect to your floors climbed goal, you can view your floors climbed history by using the Dashboard on either the Fitbit app or the Fitbit.com website:

» In the Dashboard, click the Previous icon (<) to go back one day. After you've gone back one or more days, you can also click the Next icon (>) to move forward a day.

» In the Dashboard, click the floors climbed metric. Fitbit opens the Floors Climbed screen, which displays a chart of the previous seven days of floors climbed and how they compare to your goal (see Figure 5-20). You can also scroll down to see the floors climbed from previous days, and you can click any day to see a timeline of when the floors climbed occurred during the day.

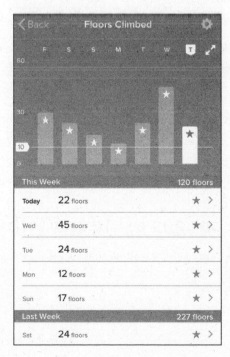

FIGURE 5-20:
The Floors Climbed screen displays your historical floors climbed data.

Achievement Unlocked: Earning Activity Badges

To help motivate and challenge you, Fitbit offers a large collection of badges that you earn by performing certain activities, such as reaching a particular number of steps in a day, surpassing a specified number of floors in your lifetime (that is, since joining Fitbit), or reaching a weight goal. Dozens of badges are available. Here's a sampling:

>> **Sneakers:** Walk or run 10,000 steps in a day

>> **Urban boots:** Walk or run 15,000 steps in a day

>> **Olympian sandals:** Walk or run 100,000 steps in a day

>> **Marathon:** Walk or run 26 miles since joining Fitbit

>> **London:** Walk or run 250 miles since joining Fitbit

>> **Pole to pole:** Walk or run 12,430 miles since joining Fitbit

>> **Happy hill:** Climb 10 floors in a day

>> **Redwood forest:** Climb 25 floors in a day

>> **Skyscraper:** Climb 100 floors in a day

>> **Helicopter:** Climb 500 floors since joining Fitbit

>> **Skydiver:** Climb 1,000 floors since joining Fitbit

>> **Satellite:** Climb 35,000 floors since joining Fitbit

>> **Weight goal met:** Reach your weight goal

>> **10-pound weight loss:** Lose 10 pounds since setting your weight goal

>> **100-pound weight loss:** Lose 100 pounds since setting your weight goal

REMEMBER

To see the full list of badges, go to `https://blog.fitbit.com/fitbit-badges/`.

Viewing your badges using the Fitbit app

To see the badges you've earned so far, follow these steps in the Fitbit app:

1. **Click Dashboard ⇨ Account.**

2. **Click View Your Profile.**

3. **Click Badges and Trophies.**

The Fitbit app displays your top four badges.

4. **Click Badge Collection.**

The Fitbit app displays every badge you've earned.

Viewing your badges using Fitbit.com

Follow these steps to use Fitbit.com to see the badges you've earned:

1. **Surf to www.fitbit.com and log in to display the Dashboard.**

2. **Hover the mouse pointer over the Badges tile and click the Next icon (>) or Previous icon (<) to navigate your top four badges.**

3. **Hover the mouse pointer over the Badges tile and click See More.**

   Fitbit.com displays every badge you've earned. Note that you can also display this page directly by heading to www.fitbit.com/badges.

IN THIS CHAPTER

» **Understanding how Fitbit tracks sleep**

» **Setting a sleep goal**

» **Tracking your time asleep and sleep stages**

» **Adding to and editing your sleep log manually**

» **Setting a wake-up alarm**

Chapter **6**

Tracking Your Sleep Patterns

The next time you see someone yawning during the day, or complaining about how tired she is, or walking around with that boy-could-I-ever-use-a-nap look on his face, ask that person how much sleep they got last night. Chances are the reply will be "eight hours." Unless people identify as an insomniac, they routinely overreport how much sleep they get, even as the symptoms of sleep deprivation multiply around them.

Why the discrepancy? For most people, the sleep knowledge gap comes because they go to bed at, say, 11 p.m. and wake up at 7 a.m., and consider that an eight-hour sleep. But they ignore the 15 minutes of reading before turning out the light, the two or three wake-ups during the night, and the 20 minutes they lingered in bed in the morning before finally getting up. In truth, that eight-hour sleep was really only seven or even six-and-half hours. Hence the yawning.

In other words, people think they sleep more than they do because they don't have an objective way to know how much sleep they really get. Fortunately, most Fitbits can help by tracking the amount of time you sleep at night, and many Fitbits can even track the stages of your sleep. In this chapter, you investigate these and other Fitbit sleep-tracking features. A (true) good night's sleep is just around the corner.

How Does Fitbit Track Sleep?

If you, like me, were initially struck by how *weird* is was that a wrist-based tracker could measure foot-related metrics such as steps and distance, you'll likely be as flummoxed as I was by the idea that your Fitbit can track sleep as well. Wait a minute, I said to myself. A Fitbit tracks movement, but sleep is the *absence* of movement. What in the name of Rip Van Winkle is going on here?

Although it seems as though sleep is a motionless endeavor, you move quite a bit during the night. Fitbit uses all that tossing and turning to track your sleep. Moreover, your Fitbit can track up to four sleep-related metrics: sleep states, sleep stages, time asleep, and sleep quality.

REMEMBER

All current Fitbit devices — except the Zip clip-on tracker and the Ace wristband tracker for kids — track sleep in some way.

Understanding sleep states

As you've probably learned the hard way, not all sleeps are created equal. Some nights if feels as though you're waking up every half hour and spending another half hour staring at the clock. Other nights you toss and turn, fidget and stretch, and throw off the covers only to snuggle back under them a few minutes later. Then there are those glorious nights where you're fast asleep a few seconds after your head hits the pillow and you don't wake up again until it's time to rise and shine in the morning.

These vastly different sleeps are all variations of what Fitbit calls *sleep quality*, which is an overall measure of how well you sleep. When you wear your Fitbit to bed (assuming it doesn't have a heart rate monitor), it tracks your movements during the night, which enables the Fitbit to detect three sleep states:

REMEMBER

>> **Asleep:** If your Fitbit detects no movement for at least an hour, it assumes you're asleep.

   If you don't move for an extended time while you're awake — for example, while you're reading a book or watching a movie — your Fitbit might log that period as sleep time. If that happens, you can remove the "sleep" from your log; see "Deleting a sleep," later in this chapter.

>> **Restless:** If your Fitbit detects a bit of movement — such as you turning over in bed — it marks that time as restless. That is, you weren't fully asleep, but you weren't fully awake.

>> **Awake:** If your Fitbit detects quite a bit of movement during the night, the device assumes you've woken up and marks the time as awake.

Fitbit devices that don't come with a heart rate monitor — such as the Alta and the Flex 2 — combine these states into a *sleep graph* that shows your overall *sleep pattern*: the number of hours and minutes you spent in each sleep state.

Checking out sleep stages

Knowing how much time you were awake or restless during the night is useful, but there's a more sophisticated way to track the quality of your shut-eye: sleep stages. A *sleep stage* is a type of sleep characterized by a particular level of brain activity and heart rate. In a typical night, everyone alternates through several *sleep cycles*, which can last up to 90 minutes. Each cycle is comprised of one or more periods spent in the following sleep stages:

>> **Light sleep:** You're asleep, but just barely, and you might even drift between sleeping and brief waking moments. It's easy for someone or something to wake you up, and your heart beat will be lower than its normal resting rate. When you first fall asleep, you usually end up in light sleep, and this stage is also usually the first period of each sleep cycle. It doesn't sound like good sleep, but light sleep plays an important role in promoting mental restoration and physical recovery. Ideally, between 40 and 50 percent of your total sleep will be light sleep.

>> **Deep sleep:** You're very much asleep and it's difficult for someone or something to wake you up. Your heart beat is at its lowest rate. Deep sleep is crucial for physical restoration, immune system recovery, and long-term memory storage. Ideally, between 15 and 25 percent of your total sleep will be deep sleep.

>> **REM sleep:** You're asleep, but your brain is active, usually by presenting you with vivid dreams. This stage causes lots of rapid eye movement (REM; hence the name) and your heart rate increases. REM sleep is important for memory storage, information processing, mood regulation, and learning consolidation, Ideally, about 25 percent of your sleep time will consist of REM sleep.

I should point out here that Fitbit also tracks a fourth "sleep" stage called awake, which is a measure of the amount of time you're awake during the night. If you're wondering what happened to the restless sleep state that I talked about in the previous section, Fitbit's awake sleep stage is a combined total of your restless sleep and your fully awake time.

A typical sleep cycle early in the night goes from light sleep to deep sleep, then back to light sleep for a bit, and finally to REM sleep. Later in the night, the sleep cycle usually alternates between light sleep and REM sleep.

Note that in each sleep stage, your heart rate changes. Not only that, but the change from one stage to another is characterized also by *heart rate variability* (HRV), which are beat-to-beat changes in your heart rate. Using your heart rate, HRV, and movement detection, Fitbit devices with heart rate monitors — such as the Alta HR, Charge 3, Inspire HR, Ionic, and Versa — can track your sleep stages.

Your Fitbit needs at least three hours of sleep data — that is, about two sleep cycles — before it can work out your sleep stages. Therefore, you won't see stages for any sleep that's shorter than three hours.

Your Fitbit won't track sleep stages if its battery is very low, so make sure your device is charged before going to bed. You also might not get any sleep stage data if you wear your Fitbit too loose, which can prevent it from reading your heart rate.

Calculating time asleep

Whether your Fitbit tracks sleep states or sleep stages, it uses that data to calculate the most important overall sleep metric: the number of hours and minutes that you were asleep during the night. Fitbit calculates time asleep by doing two things:

1. It uses your sleep schedule — the time you went to bed and the time you woke up — to determine the total amount of time you were in bed.

2. It takes the total time in bed from Step 1 and subtracts the amount of time you were awake during the night.

For example, if you went to bed at 11:00 p.m. and woke up at 8:15 a.m., you spent 8 hours and 15 minutes in bed. If you were awake for 45 minutes during the night, your time asleep was 7 hours and 30 minutes.

Your Fitbit won't recognize downtime as a sleep unless it lasts for at least an hour. Therefore, naps — that is, sleeps of less than an hour or so — won't contribute to your daily time asleep.

Figuring out sleep quality and sleep efficiency

From your sleep graph and metrics, you can get a sense of your overall *sleep quality*, which is essentially two (related) measures:

>> **Time awake:** The time you were fully awake during the night, both as a total number of minutes (and perhaps hours, if it was rough night) and as a percentage of time asleep.

>> **Time asleep:** The time you spent either restless or asleep (if you're tracking sleep states) or the time you spent in light, deep, and REM sleep (if you're tracking sleep stages). Most sleep experts recommend that this number fall between seven and nine hours for adults.

Some people combine time asleep with total time in bed to calculate an overall *sleep efficiency* score, which is the percentage of time in bed that you're actually asleep. For example, if you spent eight hours in bed and managed to sleep all eight hours, your sleep efficiency would be 100 percent. A more realistic example would be spending eight hours in bed and sleeping for seven and a half hours, which produces a sleep efficiency score of 93.75 percent.

TECHNICAL STUFF

If you want to calculate your sleep efficiency score, convert both your time in bed and your time asleep into minutes (for example, 8 hours is 480 minutes), divide the time asleep minutes by the time in bed minutes, and multiply the result by 100. An easier method is to view Fitbit's Awake percentage (see "Reviewing your sleep stages," later in this chapter), and subtract that value from 100.

REMEMBER

A sleep efficiency value around 90 percent (give or take a few percentage points) is pretty good. If your sleep efficiency is consistently over 95 percent, you're getting some solid sack time.

Setting Some Sleep Options

Before getting to Fitbit's extensive tools for tracking your sleep, you should take a minute (yep, that's all it will take) to adjust a few sleep-related settings.

Setting your time asleep goal

As with all your health- and fitness-related activities, you'll see progress only if you set measurable goals that you can work toward. However, sleep doesn't work like, say, steps or floors climbed, where it's normal to set constantly higher goals as you get more fit. That is, you're trying to get eight hours of sleep this month, nine hours next month, ten hours the month after that, and so on until you're sleeping all 24 hours of the day. Don't be silly.

Instead, you're trying to find what works best for you. Most sleep experts recommend the following ranges for nightly time asleep:

>> **Teenagers:** Between eight and ten hours.

>> **Adults:** Between seven and nine hours.

>> **Older adults (age 65 and up):** Between seven and eight hours.

Your ideal time asleep will almost certainly fall within the range for your age group, so if you're not sure what goal to set, choose a time in the middle of the range (such as eight hours if you're an adult). I talk more about healthy sleep habits in Chapter 11.

REMEMBER

Good sleep hygiene means not only getting enough sleep but also setting up a bedtime schedule — the time you go to bed and the time you wake up — that works best for you. I talk more about bedtime schedules in Chapter 11.

Setting your time asleep goal by using the Fitbit app

To set your time asleep goal with the Fitbit app, use the following steps:

1. **Click Dashboard ⇨ Account.**

2. **In the Goals section, click Sleep.**

   Alternatively, click the Dashboard's Sleep tile and then click either the Settings icon (gear) in Android or iOS or the Edit Goal icon (moon) in Windows 10.

   The Sleep Goals screen appears. Figure 6-1 shows the iOS version.

3. **Use the Time Asleep Goal control to set the hours and minutes of time asleep that you want to shoot for.**

   As mentioned, I cover setting up a sleep schedule in Chapter 11.

4. **While you have the Sleep Goals screen open, check to make sure that the Receive Sleep Insights switch is On (green).**

   Sleep insights are hints and tips that Fitbit displays based on your sleep data.

Setting your time asleep goal by using Fitbit.com

To set your time asleep goal with Fitbit.com, follow these steps:

1. **Surf to www.fitbit.com and log in to your account to display the Dashboard.**

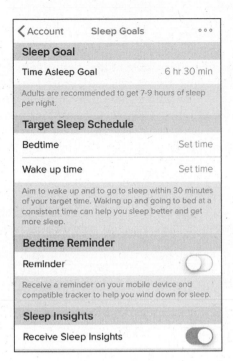

FIGURE 6-1:
Use the Fitbit
app's Sleep Goals
screen to set
your target for
time asleep.

2. **Hover your mouse pointer over the Sleep tile and then click the Settings icon (gear).**

   The Sleep tile changes to the version shown in Figure 6-2.

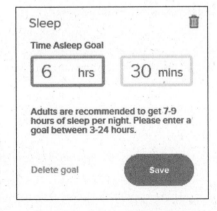

FIGURE 6-2:
Use Fitbit.com's
Sleep tile to
set your time
asleep goal.

3. **Use the Time Asleep Goal controls to set the hours and minutes of time asleep you want to shoot for.**

4. **Click Save.**

   Fitbit saves your new time asleep goal.

Setting your sleep sensitivity

One sleep conundrum you might face is your Fitbit telling you that you got a good night's sleep — say, by showing a sleep efficiency score over 90 percent — but you wake up feeling tired. What almost certainly happened is that your Fitbit underreported the number of minutes you were awake during the night. To fix that problem, you can increase the sensitivity with which your device detects your nightly movements, which will increase the amount of time it reports that you were awake.

Underreporting of awake time is a problem only for Fitbit devices that don't have a heart rate monitor. If your Fitbit doesn't have a heart rate monitor, follow the steps in one of the following two sections to increase the device's movement sensitivity.

Setting sleep sensitivity in the Fitbit app

Follow these steps to increase sleep sensitivity by using the Fitbit app:

1. **Click Dashboard ⇨ Account.**

2. **Click Advanced Settings.**

3. **Change the Sleep Sensitivity setting from Normal to Sensitive.**

   The next time you sync the app with your device, your Fitbit will apply the new sleep setting.

Setting sleep sensitivity with Fitbit.com

Follow these steps to increase sleep sensitivity via the Fitbit.com website:

1. **Head to www.fitbit.com and log in to your account to display the Dashboard.**

2. **Click View Settings ⇨ Settings.**

   The Personal Info page appears.

3. **Under Advanced Settings, click Sleep Sensitivity and then select the Sensitive option.**

   The next time you sync your device, your Fitbit will apply the new sleep setting.

Turning off notifications during sleep

If you have a Fitbit device that can receive notifications, you probably don't want to receive any alerts or messages while you're fast asleep. Good call. Follow these steps on your Fitbit device to turn off notifications when your device has detected that you're sleeping:

1. **Wake your Fitbit and display the clock screen, if it isn't displayed by default.**

2. **Swipe left to display the device apps.**

3. **Open the Settings app.**

4. **Ionic and Versa only: Tap Notifications.**

5. **Tap Off the Notifications During Sleep (Charge 3) switch or the During Sleep (Ionic or Versa) switch.**

   Figure 6-3 shows the Ionic version of the During Sleep switch.

FIGURE 6-3:
On your Ionic or Versa, tap During Sleep to Off to silence nighttime notifications.

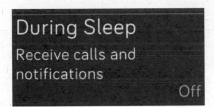

Tracking Your Sleep

Most Fitbit metrics consist of a single number: steps, floors, distance, calories, and so on. Not so with sleep, which not only offers the basic time asleep measure but also tracks your sleep schedule and your sleep stages (or states, depending on your device). Some sleep metrics also offer extra calculations such as recent averages and benchmarks, which enable you to compare your sleeps with other people of the same gender and age.

It's all ridiculously fascinating and I cover everything you need to know in the next few sections.

Tracking time asleep

The most basic — and arguably the most important — sleep metric is the total amount of time you were asleep during the night. The importance of the *time asleep metric* is reflected in the fact that Fitbit gives you many ways to track that value:

>> **Alta, Alta HR, or Flex 2:** These devices don't show time asleep, so you need to use either the Fitbit app or Fitbit.com, as I describe later in this list.

REMEMBER

On most of the Fitbit platforms, the time asleep metric is indicated by a crescent moon icon.

>> **Charge 3, Inspire, or Inspire HR:** Wake the device and then swipe up until you see the Time Asleep icon.

>> **Ionic or Versa:** Wake the device, display the clock (if it's not displayed already), and then swipe up from the bottom of the screen to open the Today app. Swipe up until you see the time asleep metric, as shown in Figure 6-4.

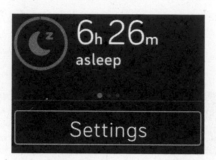

FIGURE 6-4:
Open the Today app to see this version of the time asleep metric.

>> **Fitbit app:** Open the Dashboard and view the Sleep tile, as shown in Figure 6-5. Note that this tile also includes your total awake time, a semicircle that acts as a sleep timeline displaying your bedtime and wake up time, plus your sleep stages (or states). See "Reviewing your sleep stages," later in this chapter, to learn what the different timeline colors represent.

>> **Fitbit.com:** Log in to your Fitbit account to open the Dashboard, and then view the Sleep tile.

Time Asleep icon

11:02 PM   6:13 AM

6 hr 26 min
45 min awake

FIGURE 6-5:
The Sleep tile as it appears in the Fitbit app's Dashboard.

Viewing your time asleep history

Checking out last night's time asleep is useful, but if you want to know your longer-term sleep trends and whether you need to adjust your time asleep goal, you have to check out your *time asleep history*.

Fitbit gives you three ways to examine time asleep history:

>> **Ionic or Versa:** Wake the device, display the clock (if it's not displayed already), and then swipe up from the bottom of the screen to open the Today app. Swipe up until you see the time asleep metric, and then swipe left until your see a sleep graph like the one shown in Figure 6-6.

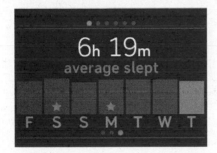

FIGURE 6-6:
The Today app's
sleep graph.

>> **Fitbit app:** Open the Dashboard and click the Sleep tile. Fitbit opens the Sleep screen, shown in Figure 6-7. The Hours Slept graph displays the previous seven days' time asleep values and how they compare to your goal. You can also scroll down to see the sleep data from previous days, and you can click any day to see more detailed data for that day (which I discuss in the next couple of sections).

>> **Fitbit.com:** Log in to your Fitbit account to open the Dashboard, hover your mouse pointer over the Sleep tile, and then click See More (or surf directly to www.fitbit.com/sleep).

Eyeballing your sleep schedule

I talk more about the importance of maintaining a regular sleep schedule in Chapter 11. For now, you should know that your Fitbit maintains a Sleep Schedule graph that you can use to get a visual indication of the consistency (or lack thereof) of your bedtimes and wake-up times.

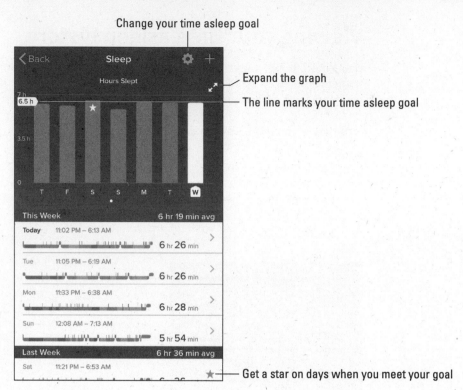

Change your time asleep goal

Expand the graph

The line marks your time asleep goal

Get a star on days when you meet your goal

FIGURE 6-7:
The Hours Slept graph displays the last seven days' time asleep values.

You use the Fitbit app to view your sleep schedule in the following two ways:

» **To see the sleep schedule history:** In the Dashboard, click the Sleep tile to open the Sleep screen, and then either swipe left on the sleep graph (Android or iOS) or click the graph's Next icon (>) (Windows 10). Fitbit displays the Sleep Schedule graph, as shown in Figure 6-8. For each day, the horizontal line represents the time you slept, so the leftmost point of the line represents the time you went to bed and the rightmost point is the time you woke up.

» **To see the sleep schedule for a specific day:** In the Dashboard, click the Sleep tile to open the Sleep screen, and then click the day you want to view. Scroll down to the Sleep Schedule section to see the sleep schedule info.

Reviewing your sleep stages

Tracking your time asleep and your sleep schedule are vital but, for my money, the real sleep tracking fun begins when you drill down into the details of each slumber to examine the sleep stages (or the sleep states, if your Fitbit doesn't have a heart rate monitor).

Bedtimes   Wakeup times

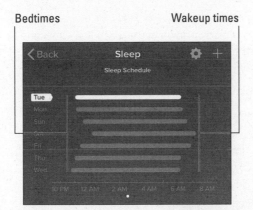

FIGURE 6-8:
The Sleep
Schedule graph
displays the last
seven days'
bedtimes and
wake-up times.

Reviewing sleep stages in the Fitbit app

To use the Fitbit app to view your sleep stages, use either of the following techniques:

>> **To see your recent sleep stages history:** In the Dashboard, click the Sleep tile to open the Sleep screen, and then either swipe left twice on the sleep graph (Android or iOS) or click the graph's Next icon (>) twice (Windows 10). Fitbit displays the Hours in Sleep Stages graph, as shown in Figure 6-9. For each of the past seven days, the different shades of blue represent the total length of time you spent in the three sleep stages: REM, light, and deep.

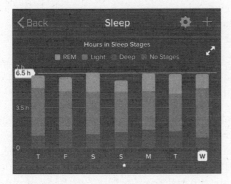

FIGURE 6-9:
The Hours In
Sleep Stages
graph displays
the last seven
days' sleep stage
totals.

>> **To see your sleep stages for a specific day:** In the Dashboard, click the Sleep tile to open the Sleep screen, and then click the day you want to view. The Sleep Stages graph (see Figure 6-10) displays a timeline of your sleep, how long you spent in each stage, and when you transitioned from one stage to

the next. You can also scroll down to the Sleep Stages section to see the time you spent in each stage (including Awake), both as an absolute time value and as a percentage of your time asleep (see Figure 6-11).

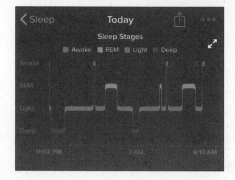

FIGURE 6-10:
The Sleep Stages graph displays a timeline of the night's sleep stages.

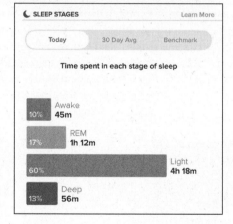

FIGURE 6-11:
The Sleep Stages section breaks down each stage by total time and percentage of time asleep.

In Figure 6-10, note that Fitbit includes a bit of awake time at the end of the sleep. Unless you're some sort of superhero who leaps out of bed as soon as you wake up, you linger a bit before you rise and, optionally, shine. Nothing wrong with that, but why does Fitbit include those last few awake minutes as part of your "sleep"? If they asked me, I'd tell them to lop off those minutes to get a more accurate sleep picture. Until Fitbit gets around to asking my opinion, feel free to mentally subtract those 10 or 15 minutes from your total awake time (especially if you're calculating your sleep efficiency score, as I describe two tips from now).

TIP

On your Sleep Stages graph's Awake line, you might see lots of tiny bars that aren't connected to the main graph. These bars represent times during the night when you woke up very briefly, often for just a few seconds.

TIP

The Awake percentage gives you a quick way to calculate the sleep efficiency score that I mentioned earlier: Subtract the Awake percentage from 100 percent. For example, if your Awake percentage is 10 percent, your sleep efficiency score is 90 percent.

Reviewing sleep stages by using Fitbit.com

Here are the steps to follow to check out a night's sleep stage data by using Fitbit.com:

1. **Log in to your Fitbit account to open the Dashboard.**

2. **Hover your mouse pointer over the Sleep tile, and then click See More.**

   Fitbit opens your Sleep log. You can also travel to your Sleep log directly at www.fitbit.com/sleep.

3. **Click the day you want to review.**

   As shown in Figure 6-12, Fitbit displays the night's sleep stage timeline and the totals and percentages for each stage.

TIP

As labeled in Figure 6-12, one bonus stat you get on the Fitbit.com display is the number of times you woke up during the night. This value includes all your brief wake-ups, so don't be alarmed if the number seems high.

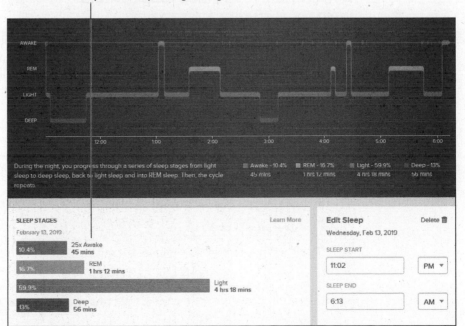

FIGURE 6-12:
The sleep stage timeline and totals as they appear on Fitbit.com.

Reviewing sleep stages on a Fitbit watch

If you have a Fitbit watch, you can view last night's sleep stage totals in the Today app. Here are the steps to follow:

1. **Wake the Fitbit and display the clock (if it's not already displayed).**

2. **Swipe up from the bottom of the screen to open the Today app.**

3. **Swipe up until you see the time asleep metric.**

4. **Swipe left.**

    The Today app displays last night's total time awake and the total time you spent in the REM, light, and deep sleep stages, as shown in Figure 6-13.

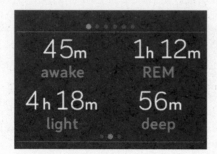

FIGURE 6-13:
The Today app displays your sleep stage totals.

Comparing your sleep stage totals with your 30-day average

Studying a night's sleep stage timeline and totals is a useful way to get a sense of how well you slept, but one night doesn't tell you much about your long-term sleep trends. Fortunately, the Fitbit app can help here by comparing a particular night's sleep stage totals with the average time you've spent in each stage over the past 30 days.

Even if you don't have 30 days of sleep data, you can still follow this procedure because Fitbit will calculate the average of however many nights are in your sleep log. Follow these steps to compare a night's sleep stage totals with your averages:

1. **In the Fitbit app, display the Dashboard and click the Sleep tile.**

    Fitbit opens the Sleep screen.

2. **Click the day you want to compare to your average.**

    Fitbit displays the day's Sleep Stages graph and data.

3. In the Sleep Stages section, click the 30 Day Avg tab.

As shown in Figure 6-14, Fitbit displays the day's sleep stage totals. For each stage, Fitbit overlays your 30-day average for that stage, designated by a vertical bar that has a dot at the bottom.

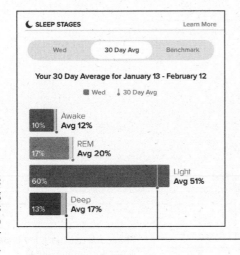

FIGURE 6-14:
The 30 Day Avg tab compares that day's sleep stages with their 30-day averages.

Bars mark the 30-day average for each sleep stage

Comparing your sleep stage totals with your peers

Comparing a night's sleep stage totals with your 30-day average is a great way to notice any changing trends in your sleep, but you might also be wondering how people like you are doing, sleep-wise. That is, how do your sleep stage totals compare with people of similar age and the same gender?

That might sound like a tough question to answer, but the Fitbit app makes it a breeze, as the following steps show:

1. In the Fitbit app, display the Dashboard and click the Sleep tile.

Fitbit displays the Sleep screen.

2. Click the day you want to compare to your peers.

Fitbit displays the day's Sleep Stages graph and data.

3. In the Sleep Stages section, click the Benchmark tab.

As shown in Figure 6-15, Fitbit displays the day's sleep stage totals. For each stage, Fitbit overlays a shaded area that represents the typical range for people of your gender and age.

How does Fitbit know what's typical for different ages and genders? It uses the data from a journal article titled (deep breath) "Meta-analysis of quantitative sleep parameters from childhood to old age in healthy individuals: Developing normative sleep values across the human lifespan." You can check it out at www. ncbi.nlm.nih.gov/pubmed/15586779.

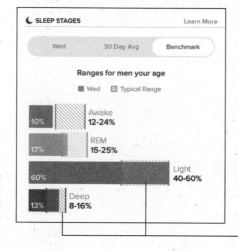

FIGURE 6-15:
The Benchmark tab compares that day's sleep stages with people like you.

Shaded areas mark the typical range for people like you

Working with Your Sleep Log

If you want to learn more about your sleep habits and tendencies, it's best to just wear your Fitbit to bed every night and let the device do its thing. That "thing" involves recording your bedtimes and wake-up times and monitoring your sleep stages (or states) throughout the night. After each sleep, your Fitbit loads all that data into your sleep log, which you can access as follows:

>> **Fitbit app:** Open the Dashboard and click the Sleep tile.

>> **Fitbit.com:** The website gives you three ways to get to your sleep log:

   ● Log in to your account to display the Dashboard, hover the mouse pointer over the Sleep tile, and then click See More.

   ● Click Log in the main navigation header, and then click the Sleep tab.

   ● Surf directly to www.fitbit.com/sleep.

Logging a sleep

What happens if you forget to wear your Fitbit one night? Well, it's not the end of the world, so you could just forget about it and move on with your life. However, if you *really* want that night's shut-eye logged, you can add it manually to your sleep log. You can't manually work with sleep stages, but you can at least record the dates and times when you went to bed and when you woke up.

Logging a sleep by using the Fitbit app

The Fitbit app gives you two ways to log a sleep manually:

>> In the Dashboard, click the Sleep tile and then click the Add icon (+) in the upper-right corner of the screen. In Android or iOS, click Add Sleep Log.

>> In the Dashboard, click the Add icon (+) at the bottom of the screen and then click Log Sleep. In Android or iOS, click Add Sleep Log.

Fitbit displays the Log Sleep screen (Figure 6-16 shows the Android version). Enter the time and date for Sleep Start and Sleep End, and then click Save.

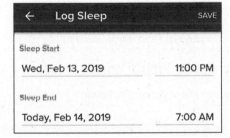

FIGURE 6-16: Use the Log Sleep screen to enter a sleep manually.

Logging a sleep by using Fitbit.com

You can add a sleep to your log by using Fitbit.com as follows:

1. Go to www.fitbit.com and open your sleep log, as described previously in the "Logging a sleep by using Fitbit.com" section.

2. In the Log Sleep section, enter the time and date for Sleep Start and Sleep End.

3. Click Log Sleep.

   Fitbit adds the sleep to your log.

Editing a sleep

If a sleep's start or end times (or dates) are wrong, you can edit them to make things right. Note, however, that you can't edit other sleep details such as sleep stages.

Editing a sleep by using the Fitbit app

Here are the steps to follow to edit a sleep by using the Fitbit app:

1. **In the Dashboard, click the Sleep tile.**

2. **Click the sleep you want to edit.**

3. **Edit the sleep entry:**

   - *Android:* Tap the Edit icon (pencil) to open the Edit Sleep screen. Type the updated times and dates for Sleep Start and Sleep End, and tap Save.

   - *iOS:* Tap the More icon (three horizontal dots in the upper-right corner). Tap Edit Log to open the Edit Log screen, type the correct times and dates for Sleep Start and Sleep End, and then tap Save.

   - *Windows 10:* Click the Edit icon (pencil) to open the Log Sleep screen. Type the new times and dates for Sleep Start and Sleep End, and then click Save.

   Fitbit updates the sleep to your log.

Editing a sleep by using Fitbit.com

You can edit a sleep by using Fitbit.com as follows:

1. **Point your browser to www.fitbit.com and open your sleep log, as described in the "Logging a sleep by using Fitbit.com" section.**

2. **Click the sleep you want to edit.**

3. **In the Edit Sleep section, enter the revised time and date for Sleep Start and Sleep End.**

4. **Click Edit Sleep.**

   Fitbit saves the new sleep data to your log.

Deleting a sleep

If you're extremely still for a long time (at least an hour), your Fitbit might think that you've fallen asleep and will add your inactive time to your sleep log. However, there might be a perfectly good (non-sleep) reason why you weren't moving for a while. For example, I've had my Fitbit record a sleep when I've been at a theater watching a movie! In that case, it's best to remove the sleep from your log to avoid cluttering it with entries that shouldn't be there.

Deleting a sleep by using the Fitbit app

Here are the steps to follow to delete an incorrect sleep from your log by using the Fitbit app:

1. **In the Dashboard, click the Sleep tile.**

2. **Click the sleep you want to remove.**

3. **Delete the sleep entry:**

   - *Android:* Tap the More icon (three vertical dots in the upper-right corner) and then tap Delete Log. When the app asks you to confirm, tap Delete.

   - *iOS:* Tap the More icon (three horizontal dots in the upper-right corner) and then tap Delete Sleep Log.

   - *Windows 10:* Click the Delete icon (trash can).

   Fitbit deletes the sleep from your log.

Deleting a sleep by using Fitbit.com

You can remove a sleep from your log by using Fitbit.com as follows:

1. **Go to www.fitbit.com and open your sleep log, as I describe in the "Logging a sleep by using Fitbit.com" section.**

2. **Click the sleep you want to get rid of.**

3. **Click Delete.**

   Fitbit asks you to confirm.

4. **Click Delete Entry.**

   Fitbit removes the sleep from your log.

Setting a Silent Alarm

In an ideal world, you'd go to bed early enough that you could wake up each morning without an alarm, daisy-fresh from getting the amount (and type) of sleep your body needs. That alarm-free experience would be nice, but here in the real world most of us need help to wake up in the morning, and that help usually takes the form of an alarm clock or, since this is the 21st century, an alarm app on a smartphone.

However, because you're wearing your Fitbit to bed anyway, why not use it as your very own wrist-based alarm clock? That's possible thanks to the Silent Alarm feature available with all Fitbit devices except the Ace and Zip. Why a *silent* alarm? The alarm uses only vibrations when it goes off, which is both a gentler way to wake up and not likely to disturb anyone sleeping nearby.

How you add a silent alarm depends on whether you're using a wristband tracker or a watch.

Setting an alarm on a wristband tracker

If you have an Alta, Alta HR, Charge 3, Flex 2, Inspire, or Inspire HR, you need to use the Fitbit app to set up a silent alarm. Here's how to do it:

1. **Click Dashboard ⇨ Account.**

   The Account screen appears.

2. **Click your Fitbit device.**

3. **Click Silent Alarm.**

   The Silent Alarms screen (Set Alarm screen in Windows 10) appears.

4. **Click Add a New Alarm (Add Alarm in Windows 10).**

5. **Set the time you want the alarm to go off.**

6. **If you want the alarm to repeat, click the Repeats switch to On (Android or iOS), and then select which days you want the alarm to go off.**

7. **Click Save.**

   Fitbit adds the alarm the next time you sync your device.

Setting an alarm on a watch

If you have an Ionic or Versa watch, you use the device's Alarms app to set a silent alarm. Here are the steps to follow:

1. **Wake your Fitbit and display the clock (if you don't see it by default).**

2. **Swipe left to display the app screens and continue until you see the Alarms app.**

3. **Tap Alarms.**

4. **Tap New Alarm.**

5. **Set the alarm time.**

6. **Make sure the On switch is activated, as shown in Figure 6-17.**

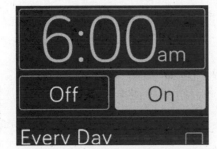

FIGURE 6-17:
Use the Alarms
app on your Fitbit
watch to add a
silent alarm.

7. **Select how often you want the alarm to run:**

   • *All days:* To run the alarm at the same time every day of the week, select the Every Day check box.

   • *Specific days:* To run the alarm at the same time only on certain days of the week, select the check box beside each of those days.

8. **Press the Back button to save your new alarm.**

Handling a silent alarm

When a silent alarm goes off, you see a screen similar to the one shown in Figure 6-18 (which comes from an Ionic watch).

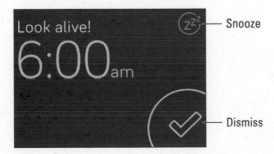

FIGURE 6-18:
A silent alarm on
an Ionic watch.

You have two ways to handle the alarm:

>> **Snooze:** To get an extra nine minutes of precious slumber, either tap the Snooze icon or ignore the alarm and it will go into snooze mode after a minute or so. If you decide to get up before the alarm vibrates again, open the Alarms app and tap the Dismiss button.

>> **Dismiss:** For a watch, tap the Dismiss icon to shut off the alarm. For a wristband, either press the device's Back button, if it has one, or double-tap the device screen.

Turning off an alarm

To deactivate an alarm, use either of the following methods, depending on your device:

>> **Wristband tracker:** In the Fitbit app, click Dashboard ⇨ Account, and click your device. Click Silent Alarm, click the alarm you want to deactivate, and then click the Turn Alarm On switch to Off.

>> **Watch:** Open the Alarms app, tap the alarm you want to deactivate, and then tap Off.

Deleting an alarm

To remove a silent alarm from your Fitbit, use either of the following methods, depending on your device:

>> **Wristband tracker:** In the Fitbit app, click Dashboard ⇨ Account, and click your device. Click Silent Alarm, click the alarm you want to remove, and then click Delete. Click OK when Fitbit asks you to confirm.

>> **Watch:** Open the Alarms app, tap the alarm you want to delete, and tap Remove at the bottom of the screen. Tap Remove again when the app asks you to confirm.

IN THIS CHAPTER

» **Understanding photoplethysmography, pulse oximeters, and other ten-dollar words**

» **Keeping an eye on your resting heart rate**

» **Tracking your heart rate during activities**

» **Figuring out heart rate zones**

» **Setting up custom heart rate zones**

Chapter **7**

Watching Your Heart Rate

Your Fitbit is mostly about measuring things that happen on the outside: the number of steps you take, floors you climb, minutes you're active, and so on. However, your Fitbit is also probably capable of internal measurements, especially your heart rate, which is the number of times your heart beats per minute. (I said "probably" in that last sentence because not every Fitbit can do the heart rate thing; of the current models, the Alta HR, Charge 3, and Inspire HR wristbands and the Ionic and Versa watches are heart-rate-friendly.) What good is it knowing your heart rate? Plenty, in fact. For example, your heart rate at rest is a good indicator of how fit you are, and your heart rate while moving is a good indicator of how hard you're working.

Your heart rate is one of the most important metrics you can track if you're serious about getting and staying fit. In this chapter, you explore how Fitbit manages the seeming miracle of getting a heart rate reading from your wrist, and you delve into all of Fitbit's heart-rate-related features, techniques, and settings.

Understanding How Your Fitbit Reads Your Heart Rate

It's slightly surprising that a device strapped to your wrist can measure steps, and it's very surprising that the same device can also tell you how much you slept last night. But it's off-the-scale surprising that your Fitbit can also monitor your heart rate. How on Earth can a Fitbit possibly figure out a heart rate?

Measuring your own heart rate is usually straightforward: You place a finger on a radial artery (located on the underside of either wrist, on the thumb side) or two fingers on a carotid artery (located in your neck, just under your jaw; one carotid artery is slightly left of center and the other is slightly right of center), wait until you feel a solid pulse, and then use a clock to count the beats for a minute (or, for the impatient, count for 30 seconds and multiply the result by 2).

Hand-based heart rate monitoring is usually the most accurate method, although it can be confounded if you use a thumb (which has its own pulse) or if you find it difficult to feel the beats. In any case, manual heart rate checking is definitely inconvenient, especially when exercising because you essentially have to stop whatever you're doing for a minute to get a reading. (Some exercisers get a quick-and-dirty heart rate measurement by doing a 10-second count and multiplying the result by 6.)

Over the years, many companies have tried to solve the problems associated with heart rate monitoring by coming up with various devices to measure heart rate automatically. Until recently, most of those solutions involved fastening a heart rate detector to your chest with a strap and then syncing the detector to yet another device — usually a sports watch or smartphone — that displays and records your heart rate.

However, strap-based heart rate monitors come with their own problems, including uncomfortable straps, flaky synchronizing, and the tendency for the detector battery to die on you mid-run.

TECHNICAL STUFF

About 20 years ago, someone came up with *photoplethysmography,* or PPG, which is a way of measuring artery volume using light. (Pronounced "foh-toh-pleth-iss-mawgruh-fee," it literally means light-based swelling measurement.) Because blood absorbs light, when you illuminate the skin with a light-emitting diode (LED), the light is absorbed if lots of blood is in the arteries under the LED or reflected back if little blood is in the arteries. That change in blood volume is caused by your heart beating, so measuring these changes is the same as measuring your heart rate. A device that both emits light and measures how much of the light is absorbed or reflected is called a *pulse oximeter.*

It didn't take long for someone else to realize that you can measure PPG from the wrist (among many other places) and that you can fit a pulse oximeter inside a watch or wristband. Voila! The *optical heart rate monitor* was born.

If you have an Alta HR, Charge 3, Inspire HR, Ionic, or Versa, your Fitbit comes with an optical heart rate monitor. To prove this for yourself, take off the Fitbit and look at the underside of the device. You'll see one or two pulsing, green LEDs: That's the business end of the optical heart rate monitor.

Beat-itude: Working with Your Heart Rate

It's eyebrow-raisingly cool that your wristband or watch can track your heart rate, but Fitbit doesn't stop at just displaying your current BPM (beats per minute). Fitbit also offers a number of other heart rate–related features, and I talk about these over the next few sections.

Checking out your current heart rate

Fitbit gives you a heartwarming number of ways to find out how fast your ticker is currently ticking:

REMEMBER

>> **Alta HR:** Double-tap the screen to wake the Fitbit. The initial screen shows your current heart rate.

On most of the Fitbit platforms, the heart rate metric is indicated by the heart icon, labeled in Figure 7-1, left.

>> **Charge 3 or Inspire HR:** Wake the device and then swipe up until you see the heart rate metric.

>> **Ionic or Versa:** You have two choices:

   ● Wake the device, display the clock (if it's not displayed already), and then tap the screen twice. Figure 7-1, left, shows the heart rate as it appears on the Ionic watch.

   ● Wake the device, display the clock (if it's not displayed already), and then swipe up from the bottom of the screen to open the Today app. Swipe up until you see the heart rate metric, as shown in Figure 7-1, middle. This screen also shows your resting heart rate, which I talk more about in the next section.

If you're out for a brisk walk or have just climbed a few stairs, you might see a heart rate metric text other than *resting* in your device's Today app or the Fitbit app (see Figure 7-1, right and left, respectively). For example, you might see the text *fat burn,* which sounds like an insult, but is actually a heart rate zone. What the heck am I talking about? See "Zoning Out: Working with Heart Rate Zones," later in this chapter.

» **Fitbit app:** Open the Dashboard and sync with your Fitbit. Your current heart rate appears in the Heart Rate tile, as shown in Figure 7-1, right. Note, too, that the Heart Rate tile also shows your resting heart rate.

» **Fitbit.com:** Your online Dashboard displays only your resting heart rate history, so see the next section to learn more.

Heart Rate icon

FIGURE 7-1:
Your current
heart rate on the
watch (left), in
the Today app
(middle), and in
the Fitbit app.

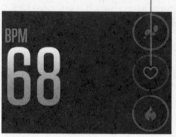 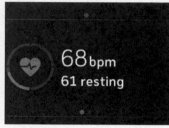 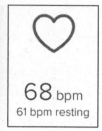

Tracking your resting heart rate

Look at the middle and right screens in Figure 7-1, and note that they both include the cryptic text *resting*. This is shorthand for *resting heart rate,* or your lowest waking heart rate, which usually occurs during the following conditions:

» You're awake (duh).

» You're sitting or lying down.

» You haven't performed any recent vigorous activity or exercise.

» You're physically relaxed and mentally calm.

» You haven't recently consumed a stimulant, such as strong cup of coffee.

» You aren't ill or taking medications that can affect heart rate.

Given these conditions, the majority of people have a resting heart rate that clocks in between 60 and 80 BPM, with most folks hovering around 72 BPM. Your Fitbit tracks resting heart rate by watching for when you are awake, are not moving, and haven't exerted yourself for a while. If you wear your Fitbit while you're sleeping, the device also uses your asleep heart rate to improve its calculation for your resting heart rate.

Resting heart rate is an important metric because it can be an indicator of health. For example, athletes and the super-fit usually have resting heart rates between 40 and 60 BPM (because the heart is strong enough to pump out more blood with each beat). On the other end of the scale (no pun intended, I promise), overweight and out-of-shape people tend to have resting heart rates well over 80 BPM, and sometimes over 100 BPM.

To see a history of your recent resting heart rate values, you have two choices:

>> **Fitbit app:** Display the Dashboard and click the Heart Rate tile. Fitbit displays the Heart Rate screen, shown in Figure 7-2, left. The chart at the top shows your resting heart values over the past 30 days. Below the chart, you see your daily historical heart rate values.

>> **Fitbit.com:** Log in to your account to display the Dashboard. Then examine the Resting Heart Rate tile (see Figure 7-2, right), which shows a graph of your resting heart rate from the past 30 days.

Expand the chart

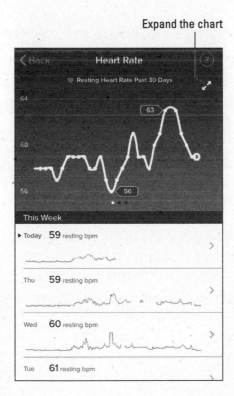

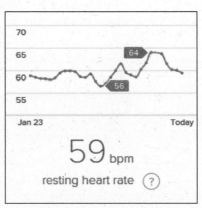

FIGURE 7-2:
Your resting heart rate in the Fitbit app (left) and on the Fitbit.com Dashboard (right).

Are Fitbit's heart rate readings accurate?

Are you wondering whether the optical heart rate monitor on your Fitbit is accurate? In a word, yes. The monitor does an excellent job of tracking your heart rate, particularly when you're at rest. In third-party measurements and in tests I've run myself, Fitbit heart rates tend to be within one or two beats per minute of a manual count or an electrocardiogram result. (An *electrocardiogram* derives super-accurate heart rates by measuring the electrical activity of the heart via electrodes placed on the skin.) Being within a beat or two isn't perfect, but it's more than close enough for everyday use.

Factors affecting heart rate

You'll almost certainly see day-to-day variations in your heart rate. Even if you always check your heart rate at the same time and same location each day, the reading can be significantly higher or lower, depending on the following factors:

>> How recently you were last active or last exercised.

>> How recently you last meditated. (Meditation tends to decrease heart rate.)

>> The ambient temperature. (Higher temperatures or higher humidity or both cause higher heart rates.)

>> Your emotional state. (Stress, anxiety, and giddiness can increase heart rate.)

>> What you've ingested recently. (Certain medications, caffeine, spicy foods, and even chocolate can raise your BPM.)

Improving your Fitbit's heart rate accuracy

Your Fitbit's heart rate reading is usually accurate, but that *usually* hedge tells you that the reading is not *always* accurate. In addition to the variability factors that I listed in the preceding section, how you wear the device can affect your heart rate readings. Here are some tips to bear in mind:

>> Always wear your Fitbit on top of your wrist.

>> When you're not exercising, position the Fitbit about one finger's width above the wrist bone (that is, towards your elbow).

>> Make sure the Fitbit is tight enough that the back of the device (where the optical heart rate monitor is located) is in contact with your skin.

If you're wearing your Fitbit but you don't see a heart rate reading, adjust the tightness of the strap (it's likely far too loose or far too tight to get a reading). Then wait a few seconds to see if the heart rate appears. If not, adjust the tightness again.

>> Make sure the device isn't so tight that it restricts blood flow under the device and messes with the heart rate signal.

>> For exercises that require frequent wrist-bending (such as lifting weights, cycling, or rowing), move the Fitbit about two finger widths above the wrist bone.

Turning off heart rate tracking

If your Fitbit's battery life is getting low but you can't charge the device right away, one solution is to use a little less power by turning off heart rate tracking. How you do this depends on the device:

>> **Alta HR:** In the Fitbit app, click Dashboard ➪ Account, and tap your Fitbit. Then tap the Heart Rate Tracking setting to Off, as shown in Figure 7-3, left.

When you're ready to resume tracking heart rate on your Alta HR, be sure to select Auto rather than On in the Heart Rate Tracking list. The Auto setting means that the Fitbit automatically shuts off the heart rate monitor when it detects it's not being worn, which saves battery power.

>> **Inspire HR:** Wake your device and display the clock. Swipe up until you see the Settings app, tap Settings, and then tap Heart Rate to Off.

>> **Charge 3, Ionic, or Versa:** Wake your device and display the clock. Swipe left until you see the Settings app, tap Settings, and then tap Heart Rate to Off, as shown in Figure 7-3, right.

FIGURE 7-3:
Stopping the heart rate monitor in the Fitbit app (left) and in Settings (right).

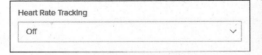

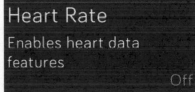

Turning off the Heart Rate feature does *not* turn off the optical heart rate monitor's LEDs, so don't be surprised if you look under your Fitbit and still see the LEDs flashing.

Zoning Out: Working with Heart Rate Zones

For many people, heart rate tracking is simple: On the practical side, they track their resting heart rate regularly, and on the fun side they watch their heart rate change as they go about their day. But if you're serious about getting fit or becoming a better athlete, you need to dig deeper into this heart rate stuff and work with heart rate zones. With these zones at hand, you can set up personal heart rate targets that enable you to get the most out of your activities and workouts, with the least risk of injury or burnout.

Determining your maximum heart rate

Before you can talk about heart rate zones, you need to know your *maximum heart rate*, which is the highest possible number of beats per minute you can achieve. Maximum heart rate depends on many factors, including your age (your maximum heart rate declines as you get older) and level of fitness (your maximum heart rate increases as you get fitter).

The standard way to calculate your maximum heart rate is to subtract your age from 220. For example, if you're 40 years old, your maximum heart rate is 220 − 40, or 180 beats per minute. This simple subtraction is the route that Fitbit takes when it estimates your maximum heart rate.

However, studies have shown that the 220-minus-your-age estimate, although close enough for most people, can be off for many folks by as much as 20 BPM either way! If you want a more accurate value for your maximum heart rate, try one or more of the following:

>> Wear your Fitbit and start running or performing some aerobic exercise. Keep the pace slow enough that you can talk out loud in complete sentences. Slowly ramp up the pace until you get to a speed where you can no longer talk fluidly — that is, you have to take a breath every few words — and then slow down until you get back to complete-sentence pace. Check your heart rate; the value you see will be approximately 70 percent of your maximum heart rate. Multiple the displayed heart rate value by 1.4 to get your maximum heart rate.

>> Take a cardiovascular stress test under the supervision of a doctor or other medical professional. This is the way to go if you're just getting started or if you have other medical issues such as heart disease or diabetes.

>> Wear your Fitbit and perform a high-intensity workout, such as running hard up a steep hill a few times. Keep an eye on your Fitbit. The largest heart rate value you see during the workout is likely pretty close to your maximum. Use this method if you're already in pretty good shape.

WARNING

The high-intensity workout route is most definitely *not* the way to go if you're out of shape or have medical issues. This type of workout is just too hard on your muscles, joints, and most importantly, your heart.

Understanding heart rate zones

After you know your maximum heart rate, you can calculate the difference between the maximum value and your resting heart rate. That difference, called the *heart rate reserve*, is a measure of, in a sense, how large a heart rate range you have to work with during your activities and workouts.

Most physiologists and trainers divide the heart rate reserve into various sub-ranges known as *heart rate zones*. Each zone is characterized by the level of exertion and how the body uses energy to power the activity.

Your Fitbit recognizes four heart rate zones and defines them by using percentages of your maximum heart rate (which, again, Fitbit calculates by subtracting your age from 220). The next few sections describe the four zones.

Out of zone

Out of zone is less than 50 percent of your maximum heart rate (for example, under 90 BPM if your maximum heart rate is 180 BPM). This zone is more of a "non-zone" because it occurs during easy activities, from resting to slow walking. Nothing is wrong with a stroll, but if you goal is to get fit (or fitter), you need to target one of the zones described in the next three sections.

Fat burn zone

The *fat burn zone* is between 50 and 69 percent of your maximum heart rate (for example, between 90 BPM and 125 BPM if your max rate is 180 BPM). Your exertion level is higher in this zone, but activities still feel fairly easy and you can carry on a conversation (assuming you're exercising with a friend).

This zone is so-named because the body tends to fuel such activities using your body's stores of fat. Specifically, any activity in this zone is fueled by using 85 percent fat, as well as 10 percent carbohydrate and 5 percent protein. Not surprisingly, this is the zone to target if you want to decrease fat, but it can also help reduce cholesterol and blood pressure.

How your Fitbit lets you know you're in the fat burn zone depends on the device. On the Ionic watch shown in Figure 7-4, left, the heart rate metric from the Today app includes the phrase *fat burn.* You see the same phrase if you have the Fitbit app nearby, as shown in Figure 7-4, right.

TIP

In Figure 7-4, left, note that the heart rate metric's circle is divided into four sections, one for each heart rate zone. As your heart rate increases and you move further into the current zone, the circle lights up to give you a visual indication of where you are in relation to both the current zone and your maximum heart rate.

Sections of the circle light as
you move into each zone

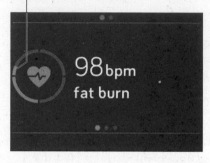
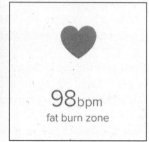

FIGURE 7-4:
The current
heart rate zone
in the Today app
(left) and the
Fitbit app.

WARNING

The fat burn zone might sound like just the ticket if one of your health and fitness goals is to get rid of some fat that's accumulated over the years. You might be asking yourself, "Why not just do all my activities and exercises in the fat burn zone?" Sticking with the fat burn zone is fine if you're just getting started on the road to fitness, but the problem with the fat burn zone is that it doesn't burn all that much fat (or expend all that many calories) because the level of intensity is on the low side. If you're interested in getting rid of some fat, you're probably better off sticking with (or building up to, if necessary) the cardio zone, discussed next.

Cardio zone

The *cardio zone* also known as the *aerobic zone,* is between 70 and 85 percent of your maximum heart rate (for example, between 126 BPM and 153 BPM if your max heart rate is 180 BPM). Cardio zone activities require much more effort and will have you breathing fairly hard. Workouts in the cardio zone are fueled typically through 50 percent fat and 50 percent carbohydrate.

Cardio is the zone to target if you want to improve your endurance, particularly your heart and lung capacity. For most folks, spending at least 20 minutes but ideally between 30 and 60 minutes in the cardio zone offers the best bang for your fitness buck.

Figure 7-5 shows how the Fitbit app's Heart Rate tile displays a heart rate within the cardio zone.

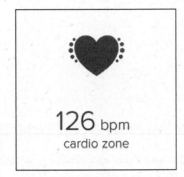

FIGURE 7-5:
The Fitbit app's
Heart Rate tile in
the cardio zone.

Peak zone

The *peak zone* is over 85 percent of your maximum heart rate (for example, over 153 BPM if your top heart rate is 180 BPM). The peak zone is also known as the *anaerobic zone* or the *threshold zone*. Activities in the peak zone are super-hard and will have you gasping for air. During activities in the peak zone, the body tends to use 85 percent carbohydrates and 15 percent fat as fuel.

A peak zone workout is designed to improve speed and the amount of oxygen you can consume during exercise, but workouts typically last only between 10 and 20 minutes. It should go without saying (but I'm saying it anyway) that you should approach the peak zone with caution and hit the peak zone only if you're already in fantastic shape.

**TECHNICAL
STUFF**

The amount of oxygen your body can consume during exercise is known in the fitness trade as your *VO2 max*. The higher the VO2 max value, the longer you can sustain a hard pace during a workout (or a race, if that's your thing). Fitbit's name for the VO2 max metric is cardio fitness score, and I talk about both VO2 max and cardio fitness score in more detail in Chapter 9.

Figure 7-6 shows how the Fitbit app's Heart Rate tile displays a heart rate that's within the peak zone.

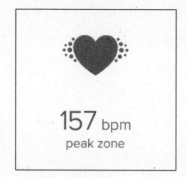

157 bpm
peak zone

Setting up custom heart rate zones

I mentioned that Fitbit's maximum heart rate calculation (220 minus your age) is fine for most people, but can be off spectacularly for others. In my own case, I know from running high-intensity workouts that my actual max heart rate is a whopping 20 BPM higher than Fitbit's calculation.

Such a drastic difference makes Fitbit's default heart rate zones useless for training. Fortunately, if you find yourself in the same boat, Fitbit allows you to customize your heart rate zones in two ways:

» **Define a custom maximum heart rate.** Keeps Fitbit's default zone percentages (such as 50 to 69 percent for the fat burn zone) but adjusts the actual zone limits based on your custom maximum heart rate. Defining a custom max heart rate is the way to go if you used any of the procedures I outlined earlier in this chapter to calculate your actual maximum heart rate.

» **Define a custom heart rate zone.** Overrides Fitbit's default zones with a single zone that you define with upper and lower limits. Defining a custom heart rate zone is the way to go if you have a specific heart rate range that you want to always target when you exercise.

You can perform either customization by using the Fitbit app or the Fitbit.com Dashboard, as described next.

Defining custom heart rate zones
by using the Fitbit app

Here are the steps to follow to define custom heart rate zones by using the Fitbit app:

1. **Click Dashboard ⇨ Account.**

    The Account screen appears.

2. **Click Heart Rate Zones (or HR Zone in Windows 10).**

    The Heart Rate Zones (HR Zones in the iOS app) screen appears and displays the lower limits for each of your current heart rate zones.

3. **To set a custom maximum heart rate, click the Custom Max Heart Rate switch to on (green), and then use the Max Heart Rate field to specify your maximum rate, as shown in Figure 7-7.**

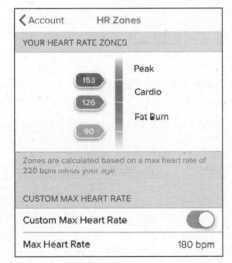

FIGURE 7-7:
Click Custom Max Heart Rate to On to set your own maximum heart rate.

4. **To set a custom heart rate zone, click the Custom Zone switch to on (green), and then use the Upper Limit and Lower Limit fields to specify the new heart rate zone's range, as shown in Figure 7-8.**

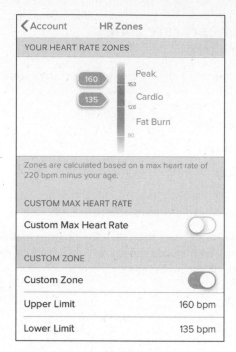

Defining custom heart rate zones by using Fitbit.com

Here are the steps to follow to define custom heart rate zones online with
Fitbit.com:

1. Surf to www.fitbit.com and log in to display your Dashboard.

2. Click View Settings ⇨ Settings.

3. Click Heart Rate Zones.

4. To set a custom maximum heart rate, select the Custom option in the
   Max Heart Rate section, and then use the text box to specify your
   maximum rate.

5. To set a custom heart rate zone, select the Custom option in the Heart
   Rate Zone section, and then use the Min and Max text boxes to specify
   the new heart rate zone's range.

6. Click Submit to save your changes.

Chapter **8**

Keeping an Eye on Your Body Composition

D o you think that most people are satisfied with their bodies? If you answered "Yes" to that question, cue the game-show "sorry, wrong answer" buzzer. Several studies over the past decade or so have shown that as few as a quarter of the population are happy with how they look. That's right: Walk into just about any room and three out of every four people you see would, if asked, have some sort of serious complaint about the way they look.

If you fall into that majority, there's a good chance you purchased your Fitbit — especially if it's an Aria 2 weighing scale — because you'd prefer to hang out with the minority who are satisfied with how they look. Whether you want to lose a few (or a lot of) pounds, maintain your current weight, or gain some weight (in the form of bigger muscles, ideally), your Fitbit can help by making it easy to track various body composition metrics. In this chapter, you explore Fitbit's tools for determining, tracking, and analyzing your body composition, with an emphasis on using the Aria 2 scale. Hop on!

What's All This about Body Composition?

"Body composition" sounds like a phrase only a tall-forehead type would love. However, it's convenient shorthand for several related measurements that have to do with your body: weight, body fat percentage, body mass index, and lean mass.

Weight

Fitbit is happy to track how much you weigh using one of three measurement units: pounds, kilograms, and stone (a wonderful British unit that's the equivalent of 14 pounds, and, yes, is always singular). You can use the Fitbit app to set up a weight-related goal, which can be to lose or gain a specified number of pounds or to maintain your current weight.

REMEMBER

You don't need a Fitbit Aria scale to track your weight. If you have a garden-variety scale at home or use a scale at the gym, you can add your weight — and your body fat percentage, if your scale detects it — to your Fitbit log by hand. See "Logging a weigh-in," later in this chapter.

Body fat percentage

Body fat percentage is the amount of fat in your body divided by your total weight. Fitbit's Aria 2 scale measures body fat percentage, as do many consumer-grade and gym-quality scales. Body fat percentage is a good indicator of overall health because too much body fat indicates obesity, which can lead to heart disease, arthritis, and other medical problems. However, too *little* body fat can also be a problem because your body needs fat to regulate temperature, keep cells functioning smoothly, protect crucial internal organs, absorb vitamins, and keep your skin and hair healthy.

According to the American Council on Exercise, here are some body fat percentage ranges to consider:

Category	Women	Men
Unhealthy (obese)	32% and over	25% and over
Average	25–31%	18–24%
Fit	21–24%	14–17%
Athlete	14–20%	6–13%
Minimum	10–13%	2–5%

How the heck can a weighing scale measure body fat? The secret is a technique known as *bioelectrical impedance analysis* (BIA). A BIA device sends a low (and safe) electrical signal up through your bare feet and into your body. That signal will readily pass through water stored in your muscle tissue, but the signal will meet stiff resistance when it encounters fatty tissue. That resistance is called *impedance* and the level of impedance is used to calculate your body fat percentage.

The electrical signal that the Aria scale sends through your body is safe for most people, but it can be problematic in some cases. For example, people with a pacemaker or other implanted medical device should not use the Aria scale (or any other body-fat measuring scale) because the electrical signal can interfere with the service. Similarly, pregnant women should also avoid using the Aria.

Body mass index

Body mass index (*BMI*) is a calculation that roughly shows your weight relative to your height. You can configure Fitbit's Aria 2 scale to display and track BMI, or you can calculate it yourself (as I describe shortly). Extremely high BMI values indicate obesity and all its related health problems, and extremely low BMI values indicate being underweight, which comes with its own health concerns. What do I mean by *extremely high* and *extremely low*? The World Health Organization offers the categories shown in the following table:

Category	BMI
Severely underweight	Less than 16
Moderately underweight	16–16.99
Underweight	17–18.49
Healthy weight	18.5–24.99
Overweight	25–29.99
Moderately obese	30–34.99
Severely obese	35–39.99
Very severely obese	40–44.99
Morbidly obese	45 and over

To calculate BMI, take your weight in kilograms and divide it by the square of your height in meters. If you don't know from kilograms or meters, divide your weight in pounds by 2.2 to convert it to kilograms, and divide your height in inches by 39.37 to convert it to meters.

WARNING

The BMI calculation works well for most people, but it can give skewed results for people with lots of muscle, such as athletes, bodybuilders, and the super-fit. The problem is that muscle weighs more than fat, so someone with a ridiculous amount of muscle will weigh a lot and thus end up with a high BMI value.

Lean mass

Lean mass (also called lean body mass) is a measurement of the non-fat parts of your body. It's the difference between your total body weight and the weight of your fatty tissue (that is, your total weight multiplied by your body fat percentage). If your goal is to lose weight, you want to make sure that what you're losing is body fat and not lean mass, so Fitbit tracks lean mass over time to make sure your lean mass metric stays more or less the same. The exception would be if you're trying to gain muscle weight, in which case you'll want to check that your lean mass is increasing over time.

Setting Up Your Aria 2 Scale

Before you can use your Aria, you have to add it to your Fitbit app and then connect the Aria to your Wi-Fi network for syncing.

REMEMBER

Technically, you don't have to add your Aria to the Fitbit app. If all you want your Aria to do is show your weight, you can use the scale as a Guest user and no setup is required.

If you haven't yet run through the setup procedure for your Aria, follow these steps:

1. **In the Fitbit app, click Dashboard ⇨ Account.**

   The Account screen appears.

2. **Click Set Up a Device.**

   Fitbit displays a list of devices.

3. **Click Aria 2.**

4. **Click Set Up (iOS), Set Up Your Aria 2 (Windows 10), or Set Up Your Fitbit Aria 2 (Android).**

5. **If you haven't done so already, pull out the plastic tab that's sticking out of the battery compartment.**

   If you've already removed the plastic tab but your Aria isn't turned on, turn the Aria over, remove the battery compartment cover, and look for the little button inside the battery compartment. Press and hold down on that button until you see the Fitbit logo on the Aria's display. Reattach the battery compartment cover.

   Your Aria displays a four-digit number.

6. **Enter the four-digit number in the Fitbit app.**

   The Wi-Fi Setup screen appears.

7. **Click Next.**

   The Select Network screen appears.

8. **Click your Wi-Fi network, enter your network password, and then click Connect.**

   Fitbit connects your Aria to your Wi-Fi network.

9. **Click Next.**

   Fitbit prompts you to select an icon that will represent you on the Aria display (see Figure 8-1).

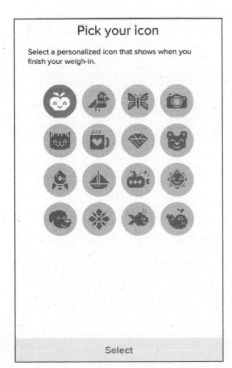

FIGURE 8-1:
Select an icon to identify you on the Aria display.

10. **Click an icon and then click Select.**

   Fitbit begins a short tutorial on using the Aria.

11. **Click Next on each screen to run through the tutorial.**

12. **At the end of the tutorial, click Done.**

   The final tutorial screen also asks if you want to add other users to the Aria. I cover adding users later in this chapter in the "Inviting others to use your scale" section.

   Your Aria is ready to go.

Setting the Aria weight unit

Fitbit configures your Aria with a default weight unit based on where you live. To check that the unit is correct or to change the unit, read on.

Setting the weight unit by using the Fitbit app

Follow these steps to set the weight unit by using the Fitbit app:

1. **Click Dashboard ⇨ Account.**

   The Account screen appears.

2. **Click your Aria.**

3. **Click Weight Units.**

   The Weight Units screen appears, as shown in Figure 8-2.

4. **Click the unit you want to use.**

   Fitbit applies the new unit setting to the Aria.

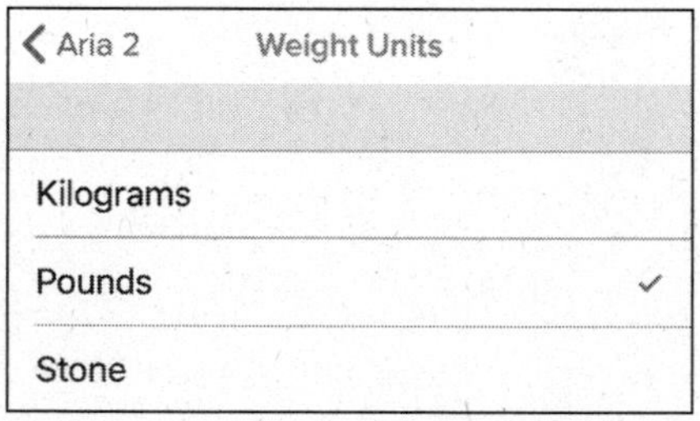

‹ Aria 2	Weight Units	
Kilograms		
Pounds		✓
Stone		

FIGURE 8-2: Select the measurement unit you prefer to use.

Setting the weight unit by using Fitbit.com

Follow these steps to set the weight unit online by using Fitbit.com:

1. **Navigate your favorite web browser to www.fitbit.com and log in to display the Dashboard.**

2. **Click View Settings and then click your Aria device.**

   The Aria device page appears.

3. **Click Scale Units.**

4. **Click the unit you want to use.**

   Fitbit applies the new unit setting to the Aria.

Configuring your Aria user settings

To make changes to your Aria user options, follow these steps:

1. **Click Dashboard ⇨ Account.**

   The Account screen appears.

2. **Click your Aria.**

3. **Click People Using This Scale.**

   The Scale Users screen appears.

4. **Click your user.**

   Fitbit displays your Aria user settings, as shown in Figure 8-3.

5. **To select a different icon, click Edit Custom Icon, click the icon you want, and then click the Back icon (<).**

6. **To toggle the display of your body fat percentage, click the Display Bodyfat (%) switch on (green) or off.**

7. **To toggle the display of your body mass index, click the Show BMI switch on or off.**

8. **To configure the scale to use lean mode, click the Lean Mode switch to on.**

   Lean mode means that the Aria adjusts how it calculates the body fat percentage to allow for people with exceptionally low levels of body fat (usually only professional athletes or extremely fit people such as marathoners, long-distance cyclists, and bodybuilders).

9. **Click the Back icon (<).**

   Fitbit applies the new settings to the Aria.

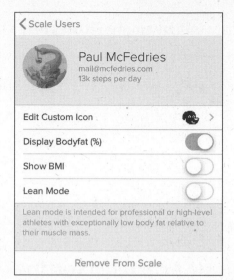

FIGURE 8-3:
Edit your Aria
user settings.

Inviting others to use your scale

Follow these steps to invite one of your Fitbit friends to use your Aria:

1. **Click Dashboard ⇨ Account.**

   The Account screen appears.

2. **Click your Aria.**

3. **Click People Using This Scale.**

   The Scale Users screen appears.

4. **Click Invite More People.**

   The Invite screen appears.

5. **Tap the Invite button to the right of the Fitbit friend you want to invite.**

   Fitbit sends the invitation to the friend.

Setting Body Composition Goals

If you're tracking your weight, it's almost certainly for a reason. For example, you want to

» Lose a few pounds.

» Maintain your current weight.

» Gain a few pounds.

Whatever the reason, you'll be far more likely to achieve your desired weight if you set up that weight as a goal in your Fitbit account. That way, you can track how you're doing relative to your goal and, if you're trying to lose weight, you can shoot for weight-loss achievement badges for extra motivation. Fitbit also enables you to set up a goal for body fat percentage.

Setting weight and body fat percentage goals by using the Fitbit app

Here are the steps to follow to set your goals for weight and body fat percentage by using the Fitbit app:

1. **Click Dashboard ⇨ Account.**

   The Account screen appears.

2. **In the Goals section, click Nutrition & Body.**

   The Nutrition & Body Goals screen appears.

3. **In Android or iOS, click Goal Weight. In Windows 10, use the Goal Weight text box to enter your goal weight, and then skip the rest of these steps.**

   Fitbit asks whether you want to lose, gain, or maintain weight (see Figure 8-4).

4. **Click Lose, Gain, or Maintain.**

   Fitbit prompts you to enter a weight goal, as shown in Figure 8-5.

5. **Adjust the weight scale to your goal weight and then click Save.**

   Fitbit asks if you have a body fat percentage goal.

6. **Adjust the body fat percentage scale and then click Save.**

   If you don't have a goal for body fat percentage, click Skip instead.

   Fitbit saves your goals and updates the Nutrition & Body Goals screen to reflect your new data, as shown in Figure 8-6.

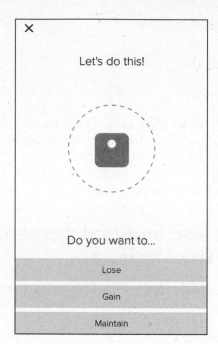

FIGURE 8-4:
Do you want to
lose, gain, or
maintain weight?

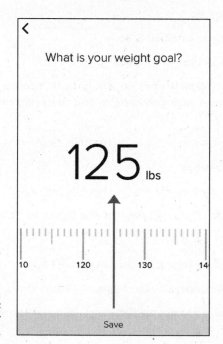

FIGURE 8-5:
Tell Fitbit your
goal weight.

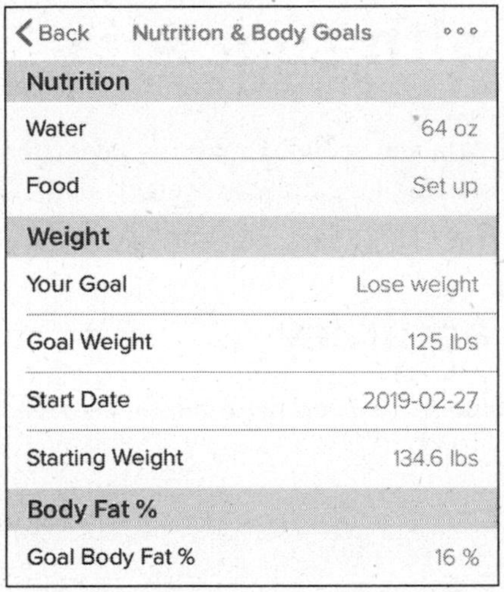

❮ Back	Nutrition & Body Goals	∘∘∘

Nutrition

Water	˙64 oz
Food	Set up

Weight

Your Goal	Lose weight
Goal Weight	125 lbs
Start Date	2019-02-27
Starting Weight	134.6 lbs

Body Fat %

Goal Body Fat %	16 %

FIGURE 8-6:
The Weight and Body Fat % sections now reflect your goals.

Setting weight and body fat percentage goals with Fitbit.com

Follow these steps to set goals for weight and body fat percentage online by using the Fitbit.com website:

1. **Tell your nearest web browser to go to www.fitbit.com, and then log in to display the Dashboard.**

2. **Hover your mouse pointer over the Weight tile, and then click the Settings icon (gear), below the Weight tile.**

3. **Click the Goal Weight tab and then click Add Weight Goal.**

   Fitbit asks whether you want to lose, gain, or maintain weight.

4. **Click Lose Weight, Gain Weight, or Maintain Weight.**

5. **Enter your goal weight.**

6. **To set a body fat percentage goal, click Goal Body Fat % and then enter the body fat percentage you want to shoot for.**

7. **Click Save.**

   Fitbit saves your goals.

Weighing Yourself with Your Aria

If you've configured your Aria and set your goals, as I describe previously in this chapter, you're ready to starting logging your weight, body fat percentage, and body mass index.

Ensuring Aria accuracy

First, here are a few pointers to bear in mind to help ensure accurate Aria measurements:

>> Place the Aria on a hard, flat surface. A soft or sloped surface might lead to wonky measurements.

>> To avoid the Aria running through frequent calibrations, try not to move the scale between measurements.

>> Weigh yourself in bare feet. The Aria can't measure body fat if you're wearing socks or shoes.

>> Make sure your feet are dry (wet or even damp feet can compromise Aria's accuracy).

>> Try to wear more or less the same thing each time you weigh yourself.

>> Try to weigh yourself at approximately the same time each day.

>> Make sure your weight is balanced between both feet after you're on the scale.

Weighing yourself on the Aria

Now follow these steps to weigh yourself on your Aria scale:

1. **Remove your shoes and socks.**

2. **Step on the scale.**

   After a few seconds, Aria displays your weight.

   If you have multiple users associated with your Aria, you might see a silhouette of a head with a question mark icon, which is Aria-speak for "Sorry, but I don't know which user is doing the weigh-in."

3. **Step off the scale.**

   Aria displays a user icon with a checkmark to the right and an X to the left.

4. **Press the right side of the scale to let Aria know the displayed icon represents you.**

   If the icon you see is *not* yours, press the left side of the scale to reject the icon. The Aria then presents the Next icon (>), and you either press the right side to accept the icon, or press the left side to reject it.

   After you accept your icon, the Aria shows your body fat percentage and body mass index (if you enabled the Display Bodyfat (%) and Show BMI options; see "Configuring your Aria user settings," previously in this chapter).

   Aria sends your measurements to your Fitbit account via Wi-Fi.

Reassigning a weigh-in to another user

When you complete a weigh-in, you might accidentally assign the weigh-in to another Aria user. That's maddening, for sure, but it's fixable using either the Fitbit app or Fitbit.com.

Reassigning a weigh-in by using the Fitbit app

Here are the steps to follow to use the Fitbit app to reassign a weigh-in to a different Aria user:

1. **Click Dashboard ⮕ Account.**

   The Account screen appears.

2. **Click your Aria.**

3. **Click Recent Weigh-Ins.**

   The Recent Weigh-Ins screen appears and displays a list of your latest weigh-ins.

4. **Click the weigh-in you want to reassign.**

   Fitbit displays the weigh-in details.

5. **In the Assign Weight section, click the user to whom you want to assign the weigh-in.**

6. **Click the Back icon (<).**

   Fitbit reassigns the weigh-in to the selected user.

Reassigning a weigh-in by using Fitbit.com

Here are the steps to follow to use the Fitbit.com website to reassign a weigh-in to a different Aria user:

1. Browse to www.fitbit.com and log in to display the Dashboard.

2. Click View Settings and then click your Aria.

3. Locate the weigh-in you want to reassign.

4. Use the weigh-in's Person list to select the user to whom you want to assign the weigh-in.

   Fitbit reassigns the weigh-in to the selected user.

Tracking Your Weight, Body Fat, and BMI

It's important to weigh yourself every day, but it's even more important to track your weight (along with your body fat percentage and BMI) over time. Unlike steps taken or floors climbed, your body composition metrics aren't under your direct control. You certainly have some input on your body composition through what you eat and how often you exercise, but the numbers that show up the next morning on your Aria are determined by how your body processes those inputs and outputs.

The upshot is that your weight tends to get away from you if you don't pay attention to it. The solution is to both perform a daily weigh-in and then track your body composition numbers over time to see your long-term trend.

Viewing your weigh-in history in the Fitbit app

Here are the steps to follow to see graphs of your historical data for weight, lean mass versus fat mass, body fat percentage, and BMI in the Fitbit app:

1. Open the Dashboard and click the Weight tile.

   Fitbit opens the Weight screen. The initial graph at the top of the screen, Weight Trends, shows your weight measurements from the past 30 days. See Figure 8-7, top left.

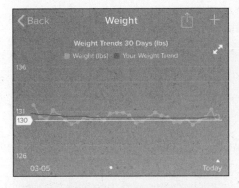
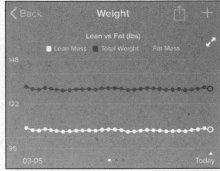
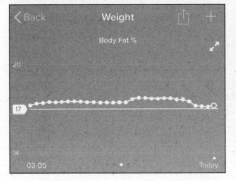
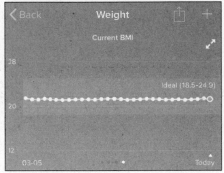

FIGURE 8-7:
The Weight
screen offers
graphs for several
different body
composition
measurements.

2. **Swipe left (Android or iOS) or click Next (Windows 10).**

   Fitbit displays the Lean vs Fat graph, which shows your lean mass (in white), your body fat (in light blue), and your total weight (in dark blue). See Figure 8-7, top right.

3. **Swipe left (Android or iOS) or click Next (Windows 10).**

   Fitbit displays the Body Fat % graph, which shows your body fat percentage values over the past 30 days. See Figure 8-7, bottom left.

4. **Swipe left (Android or iOS) or click Next (Windows 10).**

   Fitbit displays the Current BMI graph, which shows your BMI values over the past 30 days and compares them to the ideal rage for your gender. See Figure 8-7, bottom right.

Viewing your weigh-in history by using Fitbit.com

To see graphs of your historical data for weight, lean mass versus fat mass, and BMI (but not body fat percentage, for some weird reason) online by using Fitbit.com, follow these steps:

1. **Ask your web browser to display Fitbit.com and then log in to open your Dashboard.**

2. **Click Log in the navigation header, and then click the Weight tab.**

   Alternatively, surf directly to www.fitbit.com/weight.

   The Weight log appears. The initial graph at the top of the screen shows your weight measurements from the past 30 days, as well as your weight goal.

3. **Click the Next icon (>).**

   Fitbit displays the BMI graph, which shows your BMI values over the past 30 days.

4. **Click Next (>).**

   Fitbit displays the Lean vs Fat graph, which shows your lean mass (in white), your body fat (in light blue), and your total weight (in dark blue).

Working with Your Weight Log

When you weigh yourself using your Aria, the scale uploads the weigh-in data to your Weight log, which you can access as follows:

» **Fitbit app:** Open the Dashboard and click the Weight tile.

» **Fitbit.com:** The website gives you three ways to get to your Weight log:

- Log in to your account to display the Dashboard, hover the mouse pointer over the Weight tile, and then click See More.

- Click Log in the main navigation header, and then click the Weight tab.

- Surf directly to www.fitbit.com/weight.

Logging a weigh-in

If you weigh yourself while you're at the gym or out of town, you'll want to add the weigh-in data to your Fitbit Weight log to ensure the continuity of your weight data.

Logging a weigh-in by using the Fitbit app

Here are the steps to follow to log a weight and a body fat percentage (if you have one) by using the Fitbit app:

1. **In the Dashboard, click the Weight tile.**

   The Weight screen appears.

2. **Click the Add icon (+), in the upper-right corner of the screen.**

   The Log Weight screen appears (see Figure 8-8).

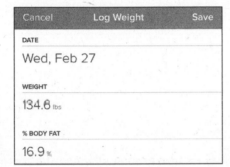

FIGURE 8-8:
Use the Log Weight screen to manually enter a weight and body fat percentage.

3. **Use the Date field to enter the date of the weigh-in.**

   In the Windows 10 version of the Fitbit app, there's no Date field, so Fitbit assumes you mean today's date. To use a different date, click the date in the Weight screen's Weight Summary section.

4. **Use the Weight field to enter your weight.**

5. **(Optional) Use the % Body Fat field to enter your body fat percentage.**

6. **Click Save.**

   Fitbit adds the weigh-in data to your Weight log.

Logging a weigh-in with Fitbit.com

Here are the steps to follow to log a weight and an optional body fat percentage online by using Fitbit.com:

1. Point your trusty web browser to `www.fitbit.com` and log in to display the Dashboard.

2. Open the Weight log, as I described earlier.

3. In the Log Weight section (see Figure 8-9), use the Weight field to enter your weight.

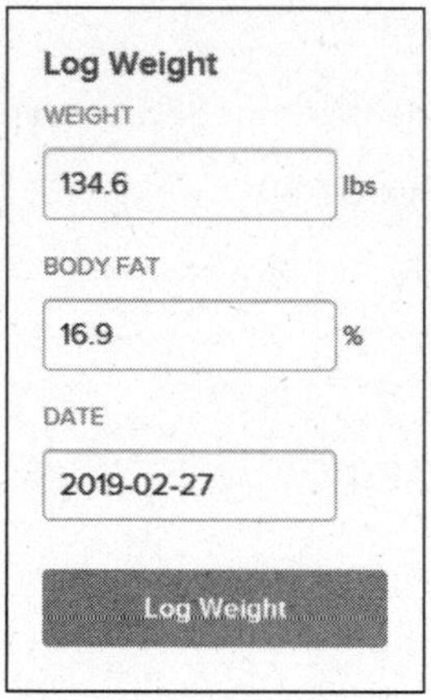

Log Weight

WEIGHT

134.6   lbs

BODY FAT

16.9   %

DATE

2019-02-27

Log Weight

FIGURE 8-9: Use the Log Weight section to manually enter a weight and body fat percentage.

4. (Optional) Use the Body Fat field to enter your body fat percentage.

5. Use the Date field to enter the date of the weigh-in.

6. Click Log Weight.

   Fitbit adds the weigh-in data to your Weight log.

Editing a manual weigh-in

If you made an error when entering a weigh-in manually, don't freak out. It's easy to fix by using the Fitbit app or the Fitbit.com website.

Editing a weigh-in by using the Fitbit app

Here are the steps to follow to edit a manual weigh-in by using the Fitbit app:

1. **In the Dashboard, click the Weight tile.**

2. **Click the manual weigh-in you want to edit.**

3. **Edit the Weight value or the % Body Fat value or both.**

4. **Click the Back icon (<).**

   Fitbit updates the weigh-in to your log.

Editing a weigh-in by using Fitbit.com

You can edit a weigh-in by using Fitbit.com as follows:

1. **Point your browser to `www.fitbit.com` and open your Weight log.**

   For details on opening your Weight log, see the opening text in "Working with Your Weight Log."

2. **Click the Edit icon (the pencil) beside the manual weigh-in you want to edit.**

3. **Edit the Weight and/or the Body Fat values.**

4. **Click Save.**

   Fitbit saves the revised weigh-in data to your log.

Deleting a weigh-in

If you have a weigh-in that you no longer need, you should remove the weigh-in from your Weight log to avoid cluttering the log and messing up your weight calculations and trends.

Deleting a weigh-in using the Fitbit app

Here are the steps to follow to delete a weigh-in via the Fitbit app:

1. **Open the Dashboard and click the Weight tile.**

   The Weight screen appears.

2. **Click the weigh-in you want to remove.**

   If you're using the Windows 10 version of the Fitbit app, right-click the weigh-in and then click Delete. You can skip 3 because you're done.

3. **Tap More (the three dots in the upper-right corner) and then click Delete Log.**

TIP

In the iOS version of the Fitbit app, you can quickly delete a weigh-in by displaying the Weight screen, swiping left on the weigh-in, and then tapping Delete.

Fitbit deletes the weigh-in.

Deleting a weigh-in with Fitbit.com

Follow these steps to delete a weigh-in online by using the Fitbit.com website:

1. **Send your browser to www.fitbit.com and open your Weight log.**

   For details on opening your Weight log, see the opening text in "Working with Your Weight Log."

2. **Click the Delete icon (trash can) next to the weigh-in you want to remove.**

   Fitbit asks you to confirm.

3. **Click Confirm.**

   Fitbit deletes the weigh-in.

3

Using Fitbit to Meet Your Goals

IN THIS PART . . .

Learn how to use your Fitbit to get in shape.

See how your Fitbit can help you lose weight.

Use your Fitbit to develop healthier habits

IN THIS CHAPTER

» **Setting activity and exercise goals**

» **Tracking walks, runs, rides, and more on your Fitbit**

» **Tracking walks and runs on the Fitbit app**

» **Viewing your exercise history**

» **Logging exercises manually**

Chapter **9**

Getting Fit

ots of people use a Fitbit to help them achieve a number of health-related goals, including getting more sleep, eating better, and reducing stress. Worthy goals all, but the truth is that most folks strap on a Fitbit because of the *fit* part. That is, their goal is to improve their overall fitness, which leads to feeling better, having more energy, a drastically reduced chance of contracting cardiovascular disease, and eating cake and ice cream without feeling guilty.

If your goal is to get or stay fit, or to improve your already-fit self, you can get there with the help of the apps and settings on your Fitbit tracker and Fitbit account. In this chapter, you explore all the fitness-related tools that are part of the Fitbit system, from setting goals to tracking exercise sessions to analyzing your workout history. By the time you've finished this chapter, you'll be ready to put the *fit* into Fitbit.

Setting Your Fitness Goals

Okay, I'm not going to sugar-coat this: If you're getting a new fitness regimen started but you don't include any concrete goals, that program will almost certainly fail. Harsh words, I know, but about a billion studies over the years have shown that people who exercise without a goal in mind almost never stick with the program. If you don't have a goal, you have nothing to shoot for, and if you have nothing to shoot for, you'll eventually stop shooting.

WARNING

If you're just starting your fitness program and you're over 50, or if you suffer from heart disease, kidney disease, diabetes, high blood pressure, or arthritis, talk to your doctor before you start doing any aerobic workouts such as running, biking, or swimming.

Although Fitbit is great at setting up goals for daily activity, it's not so good with longer-term goals. For example, if you're a runner or cyclist, you probably have weekly or monthly distance targets you want to shoot for. Fitbit can help by tracking your distance (and other metrics) over that time (see "Viewing Your Exercise History," later in this chapter), but you can't set up goals for those longer timeframes.

Setting an activity goal

Here are the steps to follow to set some daily goals for four fitness-related activities that you might want to incorporate into your fitness program:

1. **In the Fitbit app, click Dashboard ⇨ Account.**

   The Account screen appears.

2. **In the Goals section, click the Activity tab.**

   Fitbit displays the Activity Goals screen.

3. **Click Steps and then type the number of steps you want to tread daily.**

4. **Click Distance and then enter your daily distance goal.**

5. **Click Active Minutes and then type the number of minutes you want to be active each day.**

6. **Click Floors Climbed and then type the number of floors you want to ascend daily.**

7. **Click the Back icon (<) to return to the Account screen.**

   The Fitbit app syncs the new goals to your Fitbit device.

Setting an exercise goal

Fitbit defines an *exercise* as a moderate-intensity activity that lasts at least 15 minutes. You can change that time threshold, and I show you how later in the "Configuring Fitbit to automatically recognize exercises" section. For now, you can configure your Fitbit account with a goal for the number of days each week that you get in at least 15 minutes of moderate-intensity movement. Here's how:

1. **In the Fitbit app, click Dashboard ➪ Account.**

   The Account screen appears.

2. **In the Goals section, click the Exercise tab.**

   Fitbit displays the Exercise Goals screen.

3. **In the Goals section, click X Days (where X is the current goal).**

   Fitbit displays the Weekly Exercise Goal screen, shown in Figure 9-1.

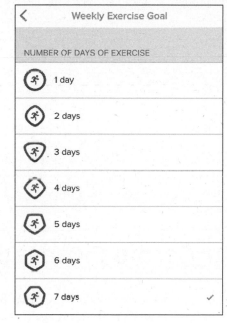

FIGURE 9-1:
Set the number of days per week that you want to perform at least one exercise session.

4. **Click the number of days per week that you want to get in at least one exercise session.**

5. **Click the Back icon (<) until you reach the Account screen.**

   The Fitbit app syncs the new goal to your Fitbit.

TIP

MAKING A WEEKLY EXERCISE PLAN

When I'm writing, say, a chapter in a book and I open a new word processing document, if I try to write with that blank screen staring back at me, I freeze. However, if instead of a blank screen I have a detailed outline of the topics I want to cover, the chapter practically writes itself.

Surprisingly, your fitness program is similar. Sure, it's great that you have daily activity goals and a weekly exercise goal, but for most people those aren't enough. They're like a blank word processing document because all you have are abstract numbers to aim for. Instead, you need to construct a kind of exercise "outline." At the beginning of each week, make a list of all the exercise sessions you intend to do. Be specific. That is, for each session, write down the following:

- Type of exercise
- Duration of the exercise
- Day of the week
- Time of day
- Location

Studies have shown that people who make a concrete weekly exercise plan are two or three times more likely to follow through on that plan than people who go into each week with a vague goal of getting in some exercise, like, whenever.

Understanding Your Cardio Fitness Score

How fit are you? That might sound like a vague question that deserves a vague answer such as "not very" or "reasonably" or "impressively." If all you have to go by are fuzzy metrics such as how much energy you have or how good you feel mentally, any answer you give to the "How fit are you?" question will be equally fuzzy. The situation improves somewhat if you try to answer the question by looking at more concrete metrics such as distance and pace. However, even these hard numbers can still tell you only how fit you are relatively (by, say, improving over time).

If you want an objective measure of your fitness — that is, a measure that tells you not only how fit you are today compared to, say, a year ago, but also how fit you are compared to people with the same gender and age range — you need to look elsewhere. That elsewhere is a metric that exercise scientists call VO2 max and that Fitbit calls the cardio fitness score.

VO2 what?

The term *VO2 max* (or, often, VO₂ max) comes from *volume* (V), *oxygen* (O₂), and *maximum* (max), and it refers to the maximum rate of oxygen consumption that occurs when a person performs exercise of increasing intensity. (This is why VO2 max is also called *maximal oxygen uptake* or *maximal aerobic capacity*.) VO2 max measures how efficiently or readily your body uses oxygen when you're exercising as hard as you can, which means it's an excellent measure of your cardiovascular (that is, aerobic) fitness.

To wit: Fit people are better able to distribute oxygen (via the bloodstream) to their hard-working muscles than less fit people, meaning they can run (or cycle or swim or whatever) faster and longer than the less fit.

VO2 max is notoriously difficult to measure and usually requires you to perform a treadmill test to exhaustion while wearing a ventilation mask that measures oxygen breathed in and carbon dioxide breathed out. The difficulty of the traditional VO2 max test is why the folks at Fitbit came up with the cardio fitness score alternative. Fitbit takes your resting heart rate, age, gender, and weight, and combines them to calculate your *cardio fitness score*, which is an estimate of your VO2 max.

TIP

People with higher VO2 max scores can run a given distance at a given speed with a lower heart rate than people with a lower VO2 max, so Fitbit can also use heart rate and GPS data from a run to calculate a more precise cardio fitness score. If you have a Fitbit with a built-in heart rate monitor and access to GPS, use the Fitbit to track a run of at least ten minutes (see "Tracking exercises on your Fitbit," later in this chapter).

Checking out your cardio fitness score

With your cardio fitness score in hand, Fitbit then slots you into a *cardio fitness level*, which tells you where you rate in relation to people of the same gender and age range. There are six levels in all: poor, fair, average, good, very good, and excellent. To see how you rate, follow these steps:

1. **In the Fitbit app, click the Dashboard's Heart Rate tile.**

   The Heart Rate screen appears.

2. **Swipe left on the graph (Android or iOS) or click Next twice (Windows 10).**

   The Cardio Fitness graph appears, as shown in Figure 9-2. A marker on the graph shows your current cardio fitness level and cardio fitness score.

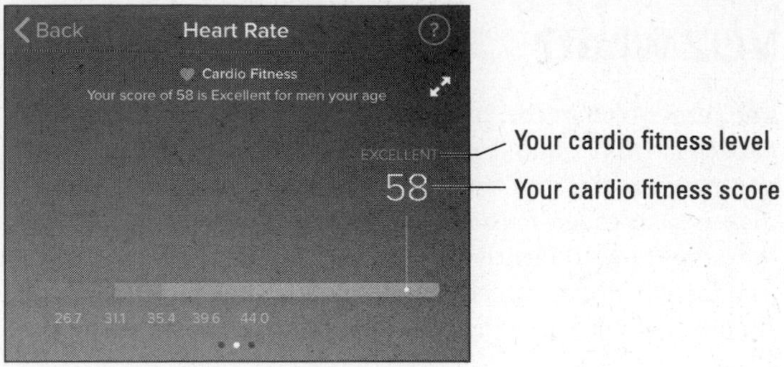

FIGURE 9-2:
The Cardio
Fitness graph
shows you
where you rate
compared to
your peers.

Improving your cardio fitness score

If your cardio fitness score relegated you to the average, fair, or even poor cardio fitness level, you should just give up, right? Don't be silly! You can bump up your VO2 max in just a few months in many ways. Here are a few suggestions:

>> If your activities and exercise sessions are low intensity, crank them up to medium intensity, meaning three METs or higher. (See Chapter 5 if you have no idea what MET means.)

>> Increase the number of weekly minutes you spend doing at least medium-intensity exercise. If you're an adult, you should be doing at least 150 minutes a week. If you're already at the 150-minute level, do more.

>> If you've been working out for at least a little while, sprinkle some high-intensity activities (at least six METs) and interval workouts into your fitness regimen. See "Setting up interval training," later in this chapter.

>> Lose some weight, especially body fat. Ideally, your goal weight should be achieved by keeping your lean mass the same (or higher), reducing your body fat percentage, and keeping your BMI in the healthy range. (For more details on concepts such as lean mass, body fat percentage, and BMI, see Chapter 8.)

Getting Your Fitbit Ready to Track Exercise

Your Fitbit can be a big part of your exercise program because it can not only track what you've done today but also show you a history of your exercises and activities. Before you get to Fitbit's features for tracking and recording exercises and workouts, you should run through a few configuration chores to make sure that your device is ready for whatever you throw at it.

Configuring Fitbit to automatically recognize exercises

One of Fitbit's handiest features is *exercise auto-recognition*, where your tracker automatically recognizes when you're doing an exercise such as a walk, run, or bike ride. Fitbit tracks that exercise for the duration and then adds it to your activities log. Sweet!

Fitbit recognizes seven modes of exercise: walking, running, outdoor cycling, using an elliptical machine, playing a sport, doing an aerobic workout, and swimming. In each case, the default minimum time it takes for Fitbit to recognize the activity as an exercise session is 15 minutes. As the next two sections show, you can customize the time for each activity.

WARNING

If you have a tracker that supports GPS, be warned that Fitbit doesn't turn on GPS for auto-recognized exercises. Because GPS gives you greater accuracy for both distance and your cardio fitness score, it's better to track the activity by using the Exercise app, which does use GPS (see "Tracking Exercise Sessions," later in this chapter).

Configuring exercise auto-recognition by using the Fitbit app

Here are the steps to follow in the Fitbit app to set up custom time minimums for Fitbit's exercise auto-recognition feature:

1. **Click Dashboard ⇨ Account.**

   The Account screen appears.

2. **In the Goals section, click the Exercise tab.**

   Fitbit displays the Exercise Goals screen.

3. **In the Auto Recognized Exercises section, click the exercise mode you want to customize.**

   Fitbit displays the controls for the selected mode, such as the Walk screen shown in Figure 9-3.

4. **If you don't want Fitbit to auto-recognize the activity, click the Auto-Recognize switch to off (the switch is no longer green) and skip to Step 6.**

   In the Windows 10 app, click Auto-Detect to Off, instead.

5. **Set the minimum number of minutes that Fitbit should wait before auto-recognizing the activity.**

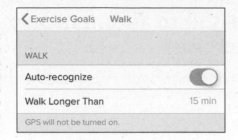

FIGURE 9-3:
You can toggle
an activity's
auto-recognition
on and off, as
well as set the
minimum
duration.

6. Repeat Steps 3 through 5 for any other activities you want to configure.

7. Click the Back icon (<) until you reach the Account screen.

The app syncs the new auto-recognition settings to your Fitbit.

Configuring exercise auto-recognition by using Fitbit.com

Here are the steps to follow online with Fitbit.com to set up custom time mini-mums for the exercise auto-recognition feature:

1. Go to www.fitbit.com and log in to display your Dashboard.

2. Click View Settings and then click your Fitbit device.

3. Click Auto-Exercise Recognition.

Fitbit displays a list of the exercises it can auto-recognize, as shown in Figure 9-4.

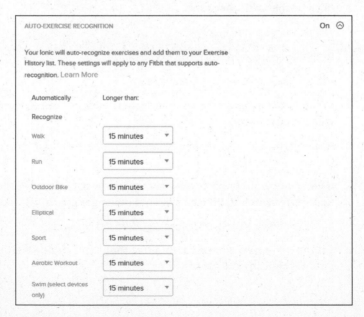

FIGURE 9-4:
The exercises
that Fitbit can
auto-recognize.

4. **Next to the exercise mode you want to customize, use the Longer Than list to select the minimum number of minutes that Fitbit should wait before auto-recognizing the activity.**

   If you don't want Fitbit to auto-recognize the activity, select Ignored in the Longer Than list.

5. **Repeat Step 4 for every exercise you want to configure.**

   Fitbit applies the new settings the next time you sync your Fitbit.

Setting up exercise shortcuts on your Fitbit

An *exercise shortcut* is a mode that appears as a separate screen in the Exercise app. The idea is that you scroll through the Exercise app screens until you find the activity you want to perform, and then select that activity. Fitbit tracks the activity for you and, when you're done, adds the session to your exercise history.

The problem is that Fitbit recognizes 20 exercise modes, but who has the time or patience to scroll through as many as 20 different screens in the Exercise app to find the mode you want? Not I, dear reader, not I. To solve this too-many-modes-too-little-time problem, Fitbit enables you to set a maximum of seven exercise shortcuts in the Fitbit app. You can also change the order of the modes, which means you can choose the seven (or fewer) exercises that you do most often, and then order them any way you want.

REMEMBER

Exercise shortcuts apply only to Fitbit trackers that can run the Exercise app: Charge 3, Inspire HR, Ionic, and Versa.

Setting up exercise shortcuts by using the Fitbit app

Follow these steps in the Fitbit app to choose and sort your exercise shortcuts:

1. **Click Dashboard ⇨ Account.**

   The Account screen appears.

2. **Click your Fitbit device.**

3. **Click Exercise Shortcuts.**

   If you don't see the Exercise Shortcuts command, it means your Fitbit can't run the Exercise app.

   Fitbit displays the Exercise Shortcuts screen. Figure 9-5 shows the iOS version.

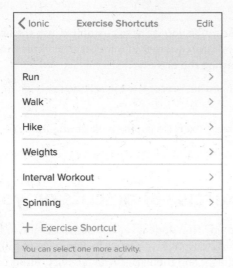

FIGURE 9-5:
Configure
your exercise
shortcuts.

4. **(iOS only) Tap Edit.**

5. **To remove a shortcut, click its Delete icon (-) and then click the Delete button that appears.**

   In Android, you delete a shortcut by swiping left on it.

6. **To add a shortcut, click the Add icon (+) and then click the exercise you want to add.**

   If you don't see the Add icon (+), it means your Fitbit already has the maximum number of shortcuts, so you'd need to delete one before you can add another.

7. **Drag the shortcuts up or down to get the order you prefer.**

   Shortcuts that appear at the top of the list appear first in the Exercise app.

8. **Click the Back icon (<) until you reach the Account screen.**

   The app syncs the exercise shortcut settings to your Fitbit.

Setting up exercise shortcuts by using Fitbit.com

Follow these steps online using Fitbit.com to select and order your exercise shortcuts:

1. **Browse to www.fitbit.com and log in to display your Dashboard.**

2. **Click View Settings and then click your Fitbit device.**

3. **Click Exercise Shortcuts.**

   Fitbit.com displays your current shortcuts.

PART 3 **Using Fitbit to Meet Your Goals**

4. **Click Edit.**

   Fitbit.com displays check boxes for every activity it can track, as shown in Figure 9-6.

EXERCISE SHORTCUTS   Edit ⌄

You can select up to seven activities

[Save] [Cancel]

☑ Run   ☑ Workout   ☑ Walk   ☑ Hike   ☑ Weights   ☑ Interval Workout

☑ Spinning   ☐ Bike   ☐ Swim   ☐ Treadmill   ☐ Elliptical   ☐ Golf   ☐ Stairclimber

☐ Tennis   ☐ Yoga   ☐ Bootcamp   ☐ Circuit Training   ☐ Kickboxing   ☐ Martial Arts

☐ Pilates

5. **To remove a shortcut, click to deselect its check box.**

6. **To add a shortcut, click to select its check box.**

7. **Click Save.**

8. **Drag the shortcuts up or down to get the order you prefer.**

   Shortcuts that appear at the top of the list appear first in the Exercise app.

   Fitbit applies the new settings the next time you sync your Fitbit.

Setting up cues

A *cue* is an update during a workout that gives you a kind of progress report. If you're running, for example, a cue might chime in every mile to tell you your total distance, elapsed time, and average pace (in minutes per mile). Having periodic reminders of how you're doing is a handy way to stay on track and saves you from having to memorize mile markers on your route, look at your watch when you reach each marker, and then calculate your pace in your head.

Fitbit offers two types of cues:

» **Lap:** A cue that's shown on the screen of your Fitbit device when you use the Exercise app to track a workout. In Fitbit land, a *lap* is a portion of your exercise session, which could be a distance (such as a mile) or a time (such as 10 minutes). This type of cue is supported by the Charge 3, Ionic, and Versa.

To learn how to configure lap cues, see "Configuring exercise mode settings," later in this chapter.

>> **Voice:** A cue that's heard on your smartphone when you use the Fitbit app to track and exercise session. To learn how to configure voice cues, read on.

Voice cues have three properties:

>> **The specific metrics output by the voice cue:** These metrics can be one or more of the following: distance, elapsed time, average pace, split pace (that is, your pace since the last voice cue), and calories burned.

>> **The frequency of the voice cues:** The frequency can either be distance-based — such as every half mile or every mile — or time-based — such as every two minutes or every 10 minutes.

>> **The volume level of the voice cues:** You have three choices: low, medium, or high.

If you track an exercise session by using the Fitbit app, you hear the app's voice cues, which use default settings: the distance, time, and average pace metrics, a frequency of every mile (or kilometer, if you've gone over to the metric side), and a volume level of medium.

Follow these steps in the Fitbit app to configure your voice cues:

1. **Click Dashboard ⇨ Account.**

   The Account screen appears.

2. **Click Exercise Tracking.**

   The app displays the Voice Cues screen, shown in Figure 9-7.

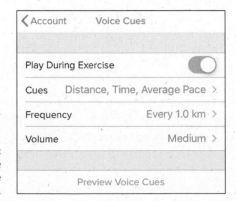

FIGURE 9-7: Configure your exercise voice cues.

3. **If you don't want to hear voice cues while you exercise, click the Play During Exercise switch to off (green isn't showing) and skip the rest of these steps.**

4. **To set the metrics output during each voice cue, click Cues, select each metric you want to include, and then click the Back icon (<) to return to the Voice Cues screen.**

5. **To set the frequency of the voice cues, click Frequency, click the distance- or time-based frequency you want to use, and then click the Back icon (<) to return to the Voice Cues screen.**

6. **To set the volume level of the voice cues, click Volume, click the level you prefer, and then click the Back icon (<) to return to the Voice Cues screen.**

7. **Click the Back icon (<) until you reach the Account screen.**

   The app syncs the voice cue settings to your Fitbit.

Configuring exercise mode settings

The exercise modes available in the Exercise app have a few useful settings that you might want to run through before tracking an exercise. You can adjust these settings by using either the Fitbit app or the Exercise app itself.

Configuring exercise settings by using the Fitbit app

Follow these steps to adjust exercise mode settings by using the Fitbit app:

1. **Click Dashboard ⇨ Account.**

   The Account screen appears.

2. **Click your Fitbit device.**

3. **Click Exercise Shortcuts.**

4. **Click the exercise shortcut you want to configure.**

5. **Configure the mode using the following settings (not all of these are available for every exercise mode):**

   - *GPS:* Ionic watch only. Toggles the use of GPS during the exercise.

   - *AutoPause:* When on, automatically pauses the exercise timer whenever the Fitbit detects that you haven't been moving for a few seconds. AutoPause is handy if you have your Fitbit inaccessibly buried under layers of clothing during winter exercising. The exercise timer resumes automatically when your Fitbit detects that you've been moving again for a few seconds.

- *Show Cues:* Select Automatic to have lap cues appear automatically according to the frequency you set in the following two settings. Select Manual to display lap cues yourself by tapping a button that appears in the upper-right corner of the Fitbit screen during the exercise; select Off to turn off lap cues.

- *Cue Type:* If you're using automatic lap cues, select the kind of lap cue you want: Miles, Kilometers, Minutes, or Calories.

- *Cue Every:* If you're using automatic lap cues, select the frequency of the lap cues.

6. **Click the Back icon (<) until you reach the Account screen.**

   The app syncs the exercise settings to your Fitbit.

Configuring exercise settings by using the Exercise app

In the Exercise app, each exercise mode offers a few settings that you can adjust to taste. To work with these settings, open the Exercise app, and swipe left until you reach the exercise mode you want to use. For the Ionic or Versa watch, tap the Settings icon (gear), in the top-left corner of the screen, as labeled in Figure 9-8; for the Charge 3 or Inspire HR wristband, swipe up to scroll through the mode's settings.

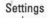

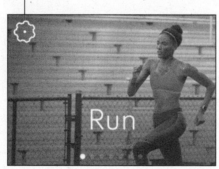

FIGURE 9-8:
Display the exercise mode you want to configure, then tap Settings.

The settings you see depend on the exercise mode, but most modes offer one or more of the following settings:

- » **Show Laps:** Determines when your Fitbit displays stats for each completed lap. There are three possible values:

    - *Automatically:* Your Fitbit displays lap stats each time you complete a lap as defined in the Automatic Lap Settings item described next.

    - *Manually:* You see lap stats only when you tap the Lap icon (oval with an upward-pointing arrow), in the upper-right corner of the screen, during the exercise.

    - *Off:* Your Fitbit doesn't display lap data.

- » **Automatic Lap Settings:** Defines a lap to use when you select Automatically in the preceding Show Laps setting. In the Lap Type option, choose a distance (Miles or Kilometers), Minutes, or Calories. In the Lap Every option, select what distance, time, or number of calories your Fitbit should use to define a lap.

- » **Customize Stats:** Determines up to three metrics to display on the screen during the exercise: one at the top of the screen, another in the middle, and a third at the bottom.

- » **GPS:** Ionic watch only. Toggles the watch's GPS on and off for the exercise.

- » **Use Phone GPS:** Versa, Charge 3, or Inspire HR only. Toggles the tracker's connection to your smartphone's GPS on and off for the exercise.

- » **Auto-Pause:** Toggles the Auto-Pause feature on and off.

- » **Always-On Screen:** When On, leaves the screen display visible during the entire exercise.

WARNING

Unless you're exercising for a very short time (say, less than 10 minutes), having your screen on full-time is a huge drain on the battery, so I don't recommend it.

Setting up interval training

In recent years, a boatload of studies have shown that one of the best exercises you can do is the *interval workout*, where you alternate periods of relatively hard effort with periods of relatively low effort (or even rest). For example, a typical interval workout would be to alternate running hard for 30 seconds and resting for 10 seconds, repeating this fast/slow pattern perhaps 10 or 15 times.

An interval workout has two main advantages: It produces results because it includes vigorous exercise, and it enables you to achieve those results relatively safely because each bout of hard effort is separated by a period — called the *interval*, hence the name of this workout — of easy or no effort. Interval workouts have been proven to produce significant improvements in cardiovascular fitness and VO2 max.

WARNING

Interval workouts are really, really tough and put quite a strain on your heart, lungs, and muscles. Don't try an interval workout if you're just getting started exercising, if you're over 50, or if you suffer from heart disease, kidney disease, diabetes, high blood pressure, or arthritis.

Your Fitbit is happy to help you track an interval workout in the Exercise app by vibrating twice at the end of each period. In Fitbit lingo, segments where you're running (or whatever) hard are called *move* periods, and the intervals are called *rest* periods. Fitbit has a default interval workout already set up for you:

>> Move period: 30 seconds

>> Rest period: 10 seconds

>> Repeats: 14

Adding up the move and rest times and multiplying by the number of repeats gives you a tough 9-minute, 20-second workout. You can customize the interval workout by using either the Fitbit app or Fitbit.com.

Setting up an interval workout in the Fitbit app

Follow these steps to use the Fitbit app to create a custom interval workout:

1. **Click Dashboard ⇨ Account.**

   The Account screen appears.

2. **Click your Fitbit device.**

3. **Click Exercise Shortcuts.**

   If you don't see the Exercise Shortcuts command, your Fitbit can't run the Exercise app.

4. **Click Interval Workout.**

   Fitbit displays the Interval Workout screen. Figure 9-9 shows the iOS version.

5. **(iOS only) Tap Edit.**

6. **Click the GPS switch to on (green) if you want to track the interval workout by using GPS.**

7. **Click Move and set the length of the move period.**

8. **Click Rest and set the length of the rest period.**

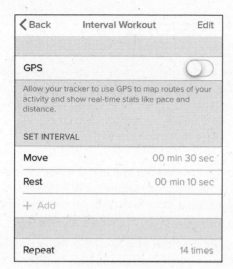

FIGURE 9-9:
Configure your
interval sessions.

9. **Click Repeat and set the number of times you want to repeat the move and rest periods.**

10. **Click the Back Icon (<) until you reach the Account screen.**

The app syncs the interval workout settings to your Fitbit.

Setting up an interval workout by using Fitbit.com

Here are the steps to follow online with Fitbit.com to set up a custom interval workout:

1. **Go to www.fitbit.com and log in to display your Dashboard.**

2. **Click View Settings and then click your Fitbit device.**

3. **If you want to track the interval workout by using GPS, click GPS and then select the Interval Workout check box.**

4. **Click Interval Workout.**

5. **In the Move text box, set the length of the move period.**

6. **In the Rest text box, set the length of the rest period.**

7. **In the Repeats list, select the number of times you want to repeat the move and rest periods.**

Fitbit applies the new interval workout settings the next time you sync your Fitbit.

Tracking Exercise Sessions

Your Fitbit automatically tracks metrics such as steps taken and floors climbed, and earlier in this chapter you discovered how to set up your Fitbit to automatically recognize activities such as runs, bike rides, and aerobic workouts (see "Configuring Fitbit to automatically recognize exercises"). However, you can get your Fitbit to track your exercise sessions in two other ways:

>> **Track the activity using the Exercise app in Fitbit devices that support it.** The Exercise app gives you access to many more exercise modes, including classes such as spinning, yoga, and Pilates; gym sessions such as weight workouts and circuit training; and sports such as tennis and golf.

>> **Track the activity using the Fitbit app.** As long as you're running the app on a mobile device (ideally a smartphone), you can use the Fitbit app to track walks, runs, and hikes.

Whether you track an exercise session by using the Exercise app on your Fitbit or the Fitbit app, Fitbit uses GPS to track your location and provide real-time pace and distance stats. GPS tracking is a big advantage over just letting Fitbit auto-recognize exercise sessions because GPS improves the accuracy of both the tracking and your cardio fitness score.

Tracking exercise on your Fitbit

If you have the Charge 3 or Inspire HR wristband or the Ionic or Versa watch, you can track a workout by using the Exercise app, shown in Figure 9-10 (this is the Ionic version).

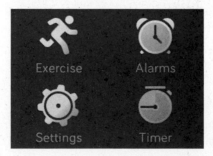

FIGURE 9-10: Use the Exercise app to track workouts on the Charge 3, Inspire HR, Ionic (shown here), or Versa.

To get started, tap the Exercise app to open it, then swipe left (or right, if needed) to locate the exercise mode you want to use, and then tap that mode.

The screen you see depends on the mode and on the Fitbit you're using. For example, Figure 9-11, left, shows the run mode screen for the Ionic watch. Note the following four items on this screen:

>> **Satellite icon:** The satellite icon and *Searching* text in the upper-left corner tell you that the Fitbit is looking for a GPS signal. You see this GPS info for modes such as walk, run, hike, and bike. For the most accurate tracking, wait until you see the *Connected* message, shown in Figure 9-11, right, before starting the session.

Set goals

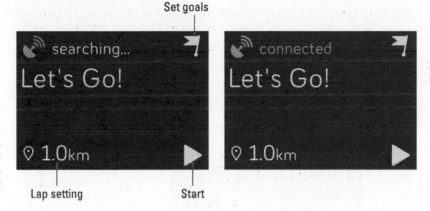

FIGURE 9-11:
The Ionic looks for a GPS signal (left) and displays *Connected* when it locks in (right).

Lap setting   Start

>> **Set Goals icon:** Tap this icon to set goals for the exercise session, such as distance or time.

>> **Lap setting:** The value that your Fitbit will use to display lap stats. See "Configuring exercise mode settings," earlier in this chapter.

>> **Start icon:** Tap this icon to begin the exercise session.

As you exercise, your tracker displays various metrics, such as distance, current pace, and elapsed time (Figure 9-12 shows a typical Ionic screen during a run). On an Ionic or a Versa watch, you can press the Back button to see other metrics, such as heart rate, average pace, and calories burned.

To pause the tracker during the exercise, use either of the following techniques:

>> **Charge 3 or Inspire HR:** Press the tracker's Back button.

>> **Ionic or Versa:** Tap the Pause icon (labeled in Figure 9-12).

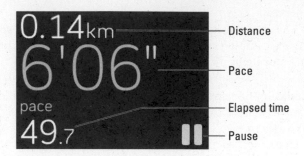

Distance
Pace
Elapsed time
Pause

FIGURE 9-12:
The Ionic screen
displays various
metrics as you
exercise.

In either case, tap the Start icon to resume tracking your workout.

To complete your workout, use either of the following techniques:

>> **Charge 3 or Inspire HR:** Press the tracker's Back button twice and then tap Finish.

>> **Ionic or Versa:** Tap the Pause icon, tap the Finish icon (labeled in Figure 9-13), and then tap End.

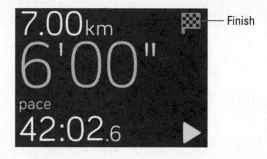

Finish

FIGURE 9-13:
To complete your
workout, tap the
Finish icon.

Tracking a walk, hike, or run with the Fitbit app

If your Fitbit doesn't support the Exercise app, or if you don't have your Fitbit with you, you can still track a walk, hike, or run by using the Fitbit app on your smartphone. Here's how:

1. **In the bottom-right corner of the Fitbit app screen, tap the Log icon (+), and then tap Track Exercise.**

   Or tap the Weekly Exercise tile and then tap the Track icon (stopwatch).

   Fitbit displays the Track screen or tab, the configuration of which depends on which Fitbit you're using. Figure 9-14 shows the Track tab that appears for an Ionic watch.

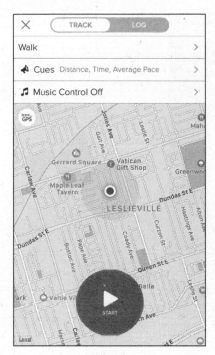

2. **Select the type of exercise: Walk, Hike, or Run.**

3. **To use voice cues during the exercise, tap the Voice Cues switch to on (green).**

   If your Fitbit supports custom voice cues, after you turn on the Voice Cues switch, you can customize the cue types, frequency, and volume.

4. **If your Fitbit supports music and you want to use the Fitbit app to control music playback during the exercise, tap Music Control and then tap the Music Control switch to on.**

5. **Tap Start.**

   The Fitbit app starts tracking your exercise and displays your progress, which includes distance, time, and pace. Figure 9-15 shows a typical screen. Note, too, that you can swipe left to see a GPS-generated map of your route and current location.

   Tap Pause at any time to temporarily stop the tracking, and then tap Start when you're ready to resume.

6. **When you've finished the exercise, tap and hold down the Finish button to complete the tracking.**

   Fitbit adds the exercise to your log.

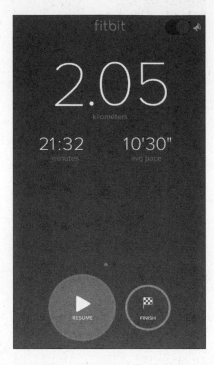

FIGURE 9-15:
During the exercise, the Fitbit app tracks your distance, time, and pace.

Working with Your Activities Log

Whether your Fitbit auto-recognizes an exercise or you use your tracker or the Fitbit app to track an exercise, everything ends up in your activities log, which you can access as follows:

>> **Fitbit app:** Open the Dashboard and click the Weekly Exercise tile. Fitbit opens the Exercise screen.

>> **Fitbit.com:** The website gives you three ways to get to your activities log:

- Log in to your account to display the Dashboard, hover the mouse pointer over the Recent Exercise tile, and then click See More.

- Click Log in the main navigation header, and then click the Activities tab.

- Surf directly to www.fitbit.com/activities.

Besides using the log to review your exercise history, you can also manually log, edit, and delete exercises, as the next few sections show.

Viewing your exercise history

One of the keys to getting in shape and improving your fitness is to slowly increase your workload. For example, if running is your fitness drug of choice, you improve fitness by slowly increasing one or more of the following:

>> Distance of your individual runs

>> Total distance you run each week

>> Number of runs per week

>> Pace of your runs

The operative word here (not only for running but for any type of exercise) is *slowly*. By a country mile, the most common cause of injury in both new and experienced exercisers is ramping up distance, frequency, or speed (or any combination thereof) too quickly.

The prudent exerciser creates a workout plan that includes modest increases each week, plus down weeks every month or two, where you drastically reduce your exercise (or even take the week off; don't worry, it'll be fine) to give your body a well-deserved break.

To ensure that you not only increase your exercise workload at a snail's pace but also take regular down weeks, take advantage of your exercise history to track your progress.

Viewing your exercise history in the Fitbit app

To check out your exercise history in the Fitbit app, display the Exercise screen, as I described earlier and as shown in Figure 9-16 (this is the iOS version).

The top part of the Exercise screen is a series of graphs that display your weekly exercise days, your monthly exercise days, your exercise durations for the past month, your exercise distances, the minutes you spent in each heart rate zone (if your Fitbit has a heart rate monitor), and your calories burned each day.

Below the graph, you see an entry for each exercise or activity. Click the exercise to see details such as your route (if your Fitbit has access to GPS), heart rate info, and calories burned.

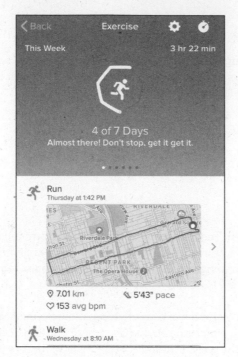

FIGURE 9-16:
Examine your
exercise history.

Viewing your exercise history by using Fitbit.com

To peruse your exercise history online by using Fitbit.com, open the activities log as I described earlier. In the Activity History section, locate the exercise you want to view and then click its View Details button. Fitbit displays the Exercise Details page, which shows exercise data such as a map and pace (if the exercise was GPS-tracked), heart rate, and calories burned.

Logging an exercise

What happens if during an exercise session you forget to wear your Fitbit and you don't bring your smartphone so you can't use the Fitbit app? If you tracked your exercise in some other way (say, by using a sports watch or stopwatch), you can add the exercise manually by using the activities log.

Logging an exercise by using the Fitbit app

In the Fitbit app, follow these steps to log an exercise manually:

1. **In the bottom-right corner of the screen, click the Log icon (+) and then click Track Exercise.**

    Or tap the Weekly Exercise tile, and then in Android or iOS, tap the Track icon (stopwatch).

2. **In Android, tap the Log Previous tab; in iOS, tap the Log tab.**

    In Windows 10, skip this step.

3. **In the Exercise Type box, start typing the mode of exercise you performed.**

    As you type, Fitbit displays a list of matching exercise modes.

4. **Click the type of exercise you performed.**

    Fitbit displays the Log Exercise screen with fields for the exercise data, as shown in Figure 9-17.

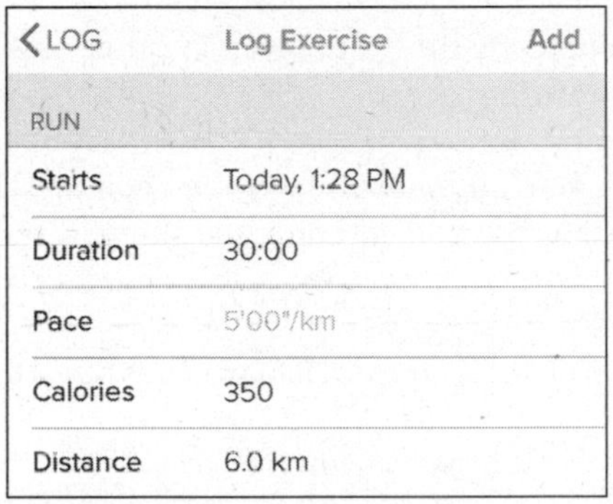

<LOG	Log Exercise	Add
RUN		
Starts	Today, 1:28 PM	
Duration	30:00	
Pace	5'00"/km	
Calories	350	
Distance	6.0 km	

FIGURE 9-17:
Use the Log Exercise screen to log an exercise session manually.

5. **Enter the exercise data.**

    The fields you see depend on the exercise, but usually include the exercise date, time, duration, distance, and calories, if known.

6. **Tap Log It (Android), Add (iOS), or Log (Windows 10).**

    Fitbit adds the exercise session to your Activities log.

Logging an exercise by using Fitbit.com

You can add an exercise to your log by using Fitbit.com as follows:

1. **Go to www.fitbit.com and open your Activities log.**

    For details, see the beginning of the "Working with Your Activities Log" section.

2. **In the Log Activities section, use the text box to start typing the mode of exercise you performed.**

    As you type, Fitbit displays a list of matching exercise modes.

    The Log Activities section also includes several default icons representing common activities, such as walking and running; you can click one of these icons and skip to Step 4.

3. **Click the type of exercise you performed.**

4. **Enter the exercise data.**

   The fields you see depend on the exercise, but usually include the exercise date, time, duration, distance, and calories, if known.

5. **Tap Log.**

   Fitbit adds the exercise session to your Activities log.

Editing an exercise

If an exercise has the wrong date, time, duration, or other incorrect data, you can edit the exercise to make things right.

REMEMBER

If you entered an exercise session manually, you can edit any of its details. If the session was tracked by Fitbit, you can edit only the starting and ending dates and times.

Here are the steps to follow to edit an exercise by using the Fitbit app:

1. **In the Dashboard, click the Weekly Exercise tile.**

2. **Click the exercise you want to edit.**

3. **Edit the exercise entry:**

   - *Android:* Tap the Edit icon (pencil) to open the Log Activity screen, enter the updated stats for the exercise, and then tap Log It.

   - *iOS:* Tap the More icon (three horizontal dots in the upper-right corner), and then tap Edit Exercise Details to open the Edit Exercise Details screen. Enter the correct data, and then tap Done.

   - *Windows 10:* Click the Edit icon (pencil) to open the Edit Exercise screen, enter the new data for the session, and then click Log.

   Fitbit updates the exercise to your log.

Deleting an exercise

If your Activities log contains an unneeded entry, it's best to remove the exercise to avoid cluttering the log with entries that shouldn't be there.

Deleting an exercise by using the Fitbit app

Here are the steps to follow to delete an exercise from your log by using the Fitbit app:

1. **In the Dashboard, click the Weekly Exercise tile.**

2. **Click the exercise you want to remove.**

3. **Delete the exercise entry:**

   - *Android:* Tap the Delete icon (trash can).

   - *iOS:* Tap the More icon (three horizontal dots) in the upper-right corner, and then tap Delete Exercise.

   - *Windows 10:* Click the Delete icon (trash can).

   The app asks you to confirm the deletion.

4. **Click Delete.**

   Fitbit deletes the exercise from your log.

Deleting an exercise by using Fitbit.com

You can remove an exercise from your log using Fitbit.com as follows:

1. **Go to www.fitbit.com and open your activities log.**

   For details on opening the activities log, see the beginning of the "Working with Your Activities Log" section.

2. **Hover the mouse pointer over the exercise you want to get rid of.**

3. **Click the Delete icon (trash can) to the right of the exercise.**

   Fitbit asks you to confirm.

4. **Click Delete.**

   Fitbit removes the exercise from your log.

IN THIS CHAPTER

» Setting a weight loss target

» Choosing a food database

» Setting up a plan for weight loss

» Logging and scanning the food
you eat

» Monitoring your weight loss plan

Chapter 10

Losing Weight

One of the unpleasant realities of using not just a Fitbit, but any fitness and health tracker, is that although a high percentage of users report improved levels of physical activity while using a tracker, a perplexingly small percentage of users report an improved diet or weight loss. For fitness and health trackers, it seems the *fitness* part resonates more strongly than the *health* part. That makes sense, in a way, because the average Fitbit is configured to make it easy to track steps taken or floors climbed. Sure, you can set up your Fitbit to track calories expended as your main goal, but when it comes to weight loss, *calories out* is only part of the equation. You also need to track *calories in,* and that's a bit more involved because it takes time to tell Fitbit what you're eating each day. And that extra time is why most Fitbit users don't use the device as a weight-loss tool.

If your goal is to lose a few pounds, this chapter shows how your Fitbit can help. Here you not only investigate Fitbit's tools for tracking your weight loss but also dig into your Fitbit account to uncarth the features and settings that enable you to log the foods you eat and easily calculate the calories you consume.

How to Lose Weight the Fitbit Way

The number of fad diets clamoring for your attention is downright mind-boggling. From the Atkins diet to the Zone diet, you can find countless weight-loss regimens as well as tens of thousands of books and websites explaining those regimens. How do you choose which one is right for you?

Two words: You don't!

Unless you have unique medical needs, a special diet is only going to make things worse in the long run (usually because starving your body of food in general or of certain nutrients in particular just makes your body retain calories and fat). Instead, all you need is your Fitbit and a commitment to the following five tasks:

>> Set a target weight

>> Weigh yourself every day

>> Log all the food and drink you consume

>> Exercise moderately (for example, by walking briskly) for at least 30 minutes every day

>> Run a calorie deficit (that is, make sure that the calories you take in are less than the calories you burn)

Yep, that's it. Study after study has shown that people who follow these simple principles are *way* more successful than serial dieters at not only losing weight but also keeping that weight off. Best of all, you can do everything with your Fitbit (including, optionally, a Fitbit Aria 2 weighing scale; see Chapter 9) and your Fitbit account.

Setting a Weight Loss Goal

You can use your Fitbit to help you keep your weight steady or even to gain weight if you're looking to pack on a few pounds of muscle. However, this chapter is about losing weight, so the first thing you should know is how to set a goal for the lower weight that you want to target. That way, you can track how you're doing relative to your goal and shoot for weight-loss achievement badges for extra motivation.

Setting a weight loss goal by using the Fitbit app

Here are the steps to follow to set a goal for your target lower weight by using the Fitbit app:

1. **Click Dashboard ➪ Account.**

    The Account screen appears.

2. **In the Goals section, click Nutrition & Body.**

   The Nutrition & Body Goals screen appears.

3. **Click Goal Weight (Android or iOS). In Windows 10, use the Goal Weight text box to enter your goal weight, and then skip the rest of these steps.**

   Fitbit asks whether you want to lose, gain, or maintain weight.

4. **Click Lose.**

   Fitbit prompts you to enter a weight goal.

5. **Adjust the weight scale to your goal weight and then click Save.**

   Fitbit asks if you have a body fat percentage goal.

6. **Click Skip.**

   Fitbit saves your goal.

Setting a weight loss goal with Fitbit.com

Follow these steps to set a goal for your target lower weight online by using the Fitbit.com website:

1. **Tell your nearest web browser to go to www.fitbit.com, and then log in to display the Dashboard.**

2. **Hover your mouse pointer over the Weight tile, and then click the Settings icon (gear) below the Weight tile.**

3. **Click the Goal Weight tab, and then click Add Weight Goal.**

   Fitbit asks whether you want to lose, gain, or maintain weight.

4. **Click Lose Weight.**

5. **Enter your goal weight.**

6. **Click Save.**

   Fitbit saves your goal.

Specifying Your Food Database

The main excuse people use to not track the food they eat is that it's just too hard. For each item of food you eat, you have to weigh it and then find out the number of calories. And if you want to track macronutrients such as carbohydrates, fat, and protein, the task is even harder.

I can't say that Fitbit solves the food-tracking problem entirely, but Fitbit does help by making it relatively easy to select a food item from a list and specify an amount. Fitbit then handles the nitty-gritty of calculating calories, carbs, and so on. Even easier is Fitbit's scanning feature, which enables you to log a food item by using your smartphone's camera to scan the food's barcode (assuming the item has a barcode).

Where does Fitbit get its list of foods? From one of its comprehensive food databases, which are specific to different countries. Food databases are available not only for the United States but also for Australia, Canada (in English and French), China, France, Germany, India, Ireland, Italy, Korea, Mexico, Spain, the United Kingdom, and more.

Fitbit assigns you a default food database according to the country specified in your account info. If you prefer a different database, or if you're visiting another country and want to track your food while you're there, you can change the database by using either the Fitbit app or Fitbit.com.

Specifying a food database by using the Fitbit app

Here are the steps to follow to specify a food database by using the Fitbit app:

1. **Click Dashboard ⇨ Account.**

   The Account screen appears.

2. **Click Advanced Settings.**

   The Advanced screen appears.

3. **Click Food Database. In Windows 10, click the Auto switch to off (not green).**

   Fitbit displays the list of countries for which it maintains a food database, as shown in Figure 10-1.

4. **Use the Food Database list to select the country food list you want to use.**

5. **Click the Back icon (<).**

   Fitbit saves your new food database setting.

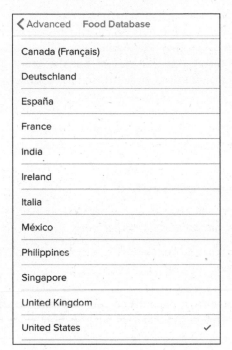

< Advanced	Food Database
Canada (Français)	
Deutschland	
España	
France	
India	
Ireland	
Italia	
México	
Philippines	
Singapore	
United Kingdom	
United States	✓

FIGURE 10-1:
Fitbit maintains
food databases
for a dozen and a
half countries.

Specifying a food database with Fitbit.com

Follow these steps to specify a food database online by using the Fitbit.com website:

1. **Cajole your favorite web browser into opening www.fitbit.com, and then log in to display the Dashboard.**

2. **Click View Settings ⇨ Settings.**

3. **Under Advanced Settings, click Food Database.**

4. **Use the Food Database list to select the country food list you want to use.**

5. **Click Submit.**

    Fitbit saves your new food database setting.

Setting Up a Food Plan

Earlier I mentioned that two of the keys to weight-loss success were logging the foods you eat and exercising regularly. These two keys represent your calories in and calories out metrics, and you can use those metrics to set up a food plan.

A *food plan* specifies your weekly *calorie deficit,* which occurs when the number of calories you consume is less than the number of calories you burn. The bigger the calorie deficit, the faster you lose weight but the more difficult the plan (because you're hungrier, more tired, or both), so Fitbit offers four different plan intensities:

>> **Easy:** A calorie deficit of 250 calories per day, which translates to 0.5 pounds (0.2 kilograms) of weight loss per week.

>> **Medium:** A calorie deficit of 500 calories per day, which translates to 1 pound (0.5 kilograms) of weight loss per week.

>> **Kinda hard:** A calorie deficit of 750 calories per day, which translates to 1.5 pounds (0.7 kilograms) of weight loss per week.

>> **Harder:** A calorie deficit of 1,000 calories per day, which translates to 2 pounds (0.9 kilograms) of weight loss per week.

Which plan intensity you choose depends on your tolerance for hunger (reducing calories in) or exercise (increasing calories out), or how close it is to swimsuit season.

REMEMBER

To help you stick to your food plan, you should set up a calories burned goal in your Fitbit account. I show you how to do this in Chapter 5.

Setting up your food plan by using the Fitbit app

Here are the steps to follow to set up a food plan by using the Fitbit app:

1. **Click Dashboard ➪ Account.**

   The Account screen appears.

2. **Click Nutrition & Body.**

   The Nutrition & Body Goals screen appears.

3. **Under Nutrition, click Food Plan (Android) or Food (iOS and Windows 10).**

4. **(iOS only) Tap Help Me Set a Goal.**

   Fitbit displays your current weight and your goal weight.

5. **If you didn't set a goal weight earlier, enter your target weight in the Goal Weight text box and then click Next.**

   Fitbit displays the Plan Intensity screen, shown in Figure 10-2.

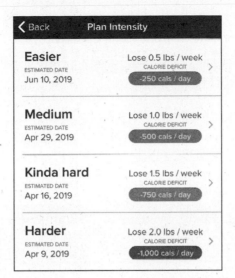

FIGURE 10-2:
Fitbit asks you to choose a plan intensity.

6. **Click the intensity of the plan you want to follow. In the Android app, tap Next.**

   Fitbit displays an overview of how it calculates its estimate of your daily calorie intake.

7. **Click Next.**

   Fitbit displays an overview of how it calculates your daily calorie deficit.

8. **Click Next.**

   Fitbit displays an overview of your food plan.

9. **Click Save Plan (Android), Done (iOS), or Save (Windows 10).**

   Fitbit saves your new food plan.

Setting up your food plan with Fitbit.com

Follow these steps to set up a food plan online by using the Fitbit.com website:

1. **Steer your browser to www.fitbit.com, and then log in to display the Dashboard.**

2. **In the Food Plan tile, click Start Now.**

   Fitbit displays your current weight and your goal weight.

3. **If you didn't set a goal weight earlier, enter your target weight in the I Want to Weigh text box and then click Next.**

4. **In the Set Up a Food Plan? section, click Get Started.**

   Fitbit displays the Plan Intensity window. To see the details of each plan, click the Show All 4 link (see Figure 10-3).

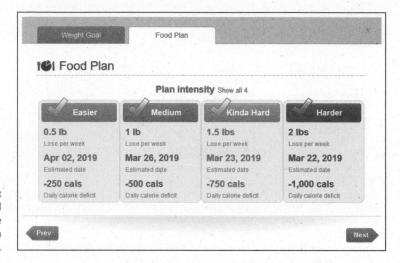

5. **Click the intensity of the plan you want to follow, and then click Next.**

   Fitbit displays an overview of how it calculates its estimate of your daily calorie intake.

6. **Click Next.**

   Fitbit displays an overview of how it calculates your daily calorie deficit.

7. **Click Next.**

   Fitbit displays an overview of your food plan.

8. **Click Next.**

   Fitbit saves your new food plan.

Logging the Food You Eat

You probably already use your Fitbit to track steps taken, floors climbed, active minutes, and exercises. These and other tracked activities contribute to the calories you burn during the day. To calculate your calorie deficit and therefore track how closely you're sticking to your food plan, you also need to tell Fitbit about the calories you ingest during the day.

Unfortunately, although your Fitbit is smart enough to determine your calories expended automatically based on your metabolism and activities, the tracker doesn't have a way to automatically track the foods you eat. Logging your food is a manual task. But thanks to Fitbit's extensive food database, it's a task that's not quite as onerous as you might think.

Accessing your food log

When you tell Fitbit a food item you've eaten, Fitbit tosses that tidbit into your food log, which you can access as follows:

REMEMBER

» **Fitbit app:** Open the Dashboard and click the Food Plan tile. Fitbit opens the Food screen.

In all Fitbit platforms, the icon for the Food Plan tile is a knife and fork sitting on a circular plate.

» **Fitbit.com:** Use any of the following to open your food log:

- Log in to your account to display the Dashboard, hover the mouse pointer over the Food Plan tile, and then click See More.

- Click Log in the main navigation header, and then click the Food tab.

- Surf directly to www.fitbit.com/foods/log.

Besides using the log to review your foods, you can also add, edit, and delete foods, as the next few sections show.

Logging food by using the Fitbit app

In the Fitbit app, follow these steps to log a food item:

1. **In the bottom-right corner of the screen, click the Log icon (+) and then click Log Food.**

Or tap the Food Plan tile and then tap the Add icon (+).

The Log Food screen appears.

2. **Locate the food item you want to log:**

- *Search:* For most food items (especially when you're just started out with food logging), you'll use the Search feature to type the food you want to log. As you type, Fitbit displays a list of matching food items, so click the item you want to log when it appears in the list.

- *Frequent:* Click this tab to choose a food item from a list of those foods you've logged most often.

- *Recent:* Click this tab to choose a food item from a list of those foods you've logged most recently.

- *Custom:* Click this tab if the food you want to log isn't in the Fitbit database. Click Add Custom Food, enter the food name (and brand, if you want), the serving size, and the calories. To add other data (such as amounts for protein, carbs, and fat), click Switch to Detailed View (or, in the Android app, click Simplified View to Off), and then enter whatever data you have. You can then skip the rest of these steps.

If Fitbit doesn't have a particular food item, you might be able to Google the item because the Google search engine has access to over a thousand food items with nutrition info. Run a search similar to *nutrient* in *food*, where *nutrient* is calories, carbs, fat, or protein, and *food* is the food item you want to check. For example, you might type calories in rutabaga.

- *Meals:* Click this tab (which, as I write this, is available only in the Windows 10 version of the app) to enter an entire meal's worth of food items, which is useful if it's a meal you eat regularly. Click Create Custom Meal, name the meal, and then add all the meal's food items. You can skip the rest of these steps.

Fitbit displays the Add Food screen shown in Figure 10-4, which you use to enter the food item's specifics.

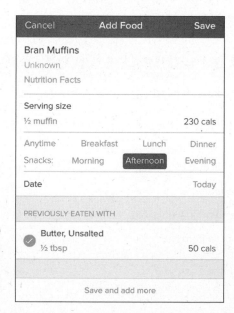

FIGURE 10-4:
Use the Add Food screen to log a food item in the Fitbit app.

3. **In the Serving Size section, specify the serving size of the food item.**

4. **Click the meal (Breakfast, Lunch, or Dinner) or time (Morning, Afternoon, Evening, or Anytime) when you ate the item.**

5. **If you consumed the item on a previous day, use the Date field to select the day.**

6. **In the Previously Eaten With section, select any item that you consumed with the item you selected in Step 2.**

   You see the Previously Eaten With section (see Figure 10-4) only if you previously logged one or more food items along with the item you chose in Step 3.

7. **To save the food item and add another, click Save and Add More, and then repeat Steps 2 through 6.**

8. **When you've finished logging foods, click Save.**

   Fitbit adds the food to your food log.

Logging food with Fitbit.com

You can add food to your log online by using Fitbit.com as follows:

1. **Go to www.fitbit.com and open your food log.**

   For details, see the "Accessing your food log" section, previously in the chapter.

2. **Locate the food item you want to log:**

   - *What Did You Eat?:* For most food items (especially when you're just starting out with food logging), you enter the food you want to log by using the What Did You Eat? box (in the Food Log section; see Figure 10-5). As you type, Fitbit displays a list of matching food items, so click the item you want to log when it shows up in the list.

   - *Most Logged:* Click this tab (in the Foods sidebar) to choose a food item from a list of those foods you've logged most often.

   - *Recent:* Click this tab (in the Foods sidebar) to choose a food item from a list of those foods you've logged most recently.

   - *Foods:* Use this tab in the Favorites sidebar if the food you want to log isn't in the Fitbit database. Click Create a New Food, and enter the food name (and brand, if you want), the serving size, and then the calories. To add other data (such as amounts for protein, carbs, and fat), click Add Nutritional Information, and then enter whatever data you have. You can skip the rest of these steps.

TIP

To add a logged food item to the Favorites tab, locate the item in the Logged Foods section and then click the item's star in the Fav column.

- *Meals:* Use this tab in the Favorites sidebar to enter an entire meal's worth of food items, which is useful if you eat the meal regularly. Click Create a Meal, name the meal, click Save, and then add all the meal's food items. You can skip the rest of these steps.

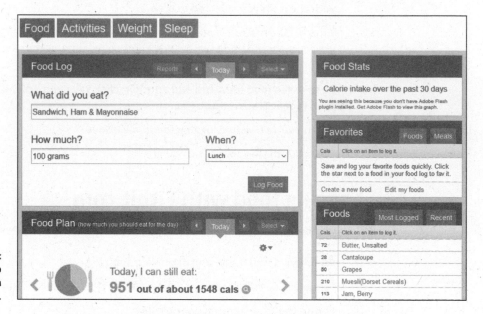

FIGURE 10-5:
Use the Food tab to log a food item using Fitbit.com.

3. **In the How Much? section, specify the serving size of the food item.**

4. **Use the When? list to select the meal (Breakfast, Lunch, or Dinner) or time (Morning Snack, Afternoon Snack, After Dinner, or Anytime) when you ate the item.**

5. **If you consumed the item on a previous day, use the Date field to select the day.**

6. **Click Log Food.**

   Fitbit adds the food to your food log.

Scanning food by using the Fitbit app

Weighing and measuring food items is nobody's idea of a good time, but it's an inevitable part of the food logging process. However, it doesn't have to be the only way you log food. If the food item comes with a barcode, you can use your smartphone's camera and the Fitbit app to scan that code and enter all the details automatically. It's a sweet feature and it works like this:

1. **In the bottom-right corner of the Fitbit screen, click the Log icon (+), and then click Log Food.**

   Or tap the Food Plan tile and then tap the Add icon (+).

   The Log Food screen appears.

2. **Click the Barcode icon, which appears near the top of the screen in Android and iOS (see Figure 10-6) and at the bottom of the screen in Windows 10.**

   Fitbit brings up your smartphone's back camera and displays a frame marked by its four corners.

FIGURE 10-6:
Click the Barcode
icon to scan a
food item.

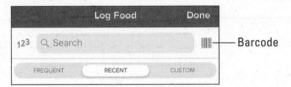
Barcode

3. **Center the food item's barcode within the frame, as shown in Figure 10-7.**

   When the frame corners turn green, Fitbit has found the barcode and grabbed the food's info. The Log Food screen appears.

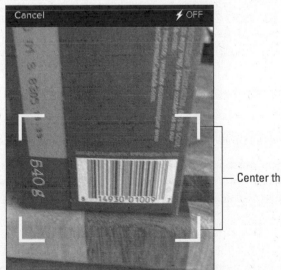
Center the barcode within this frame

FIGURE 10-7:
Center the food
item's barcode
within the frame.

4. **Make any necessary adjustments to the food data.**

   You shouldn't need to change anything here. One possible exception is serving size, which might be significantly smaller or larger than the amount you ate.

5. **To save the food item and add another, click Save and Add More, and then repeat Steps 3 through 5.**

6. **When you've finished scanning foods, click Save.**

   Fitbit adds the food to your food log.

Editing a logged food item

If you made an error when logging a food item, all is well because it's easily fixed by using the Fitbit app or the Fitbit.com website.

Editing a logged food item by using the Fitbit app

Here are the steps to follow to edit a logged food item by using the Fitbit app:

1. **In the Dashboard, click the Food Plan tile.**

2. **Click the food item you want to edit.**

3. **Edit the serving size, time, or date.**

4. **Click the Back icon (<).**

   Fitbit updates the weigh-in to your log.

Editing a logged food item by using Fitbit.com

You can edit a logged food item's amount and time slot by using Fitbit.com as follows:

1. **Send your browser to `www.fitbit.com`, and open your food log.**

   For details, see the "Accessing your food log" section, earlier in the chapter.

2. **In the Logged Foods section, edit the food item's serving size.**

3. **If you enter the food into the wrong time slot, move the mouse pointer over the item (but not over any of the item's links) and then drag and drop the item inside the correct time slot.**

   Fitbit saves the revised food data to your log.

Deleting a logged food item

If you have a logged food item that you no longer need, you should remove the item from your food log to avoid cluttering the log and messing up your calorie calculations.

Deleting a logged food item by using the Fitbit app

Here are the steps to follow to delete a logged food item by using the Fitbit app:

- » **iOS:** Display the Food screen, swipe left on the item, and then tap Delete.

- » **Android:** Open the Dashboard and click the Food Plan tile. Then click the logged food item you want to remove, tap the More icon (three dots), and then click Delete Log.

- » **Windows 10:** Open the Dashboard and click the Food Plan tile. Then right-click the logged food item and click Delete.

Deleting a logged food item with Fitbit.com

Follow these steps to delete a food item online by using the Fitbit.com website:

1. Dispatch your browser to www.fitbit.com, and open your food log.

   For details, see the "Accessing your food log" section, previously in the chapter.

2. Hover the mouse pointer over the logged food item you want to remove.

3. Click the Delete (X) icon that appears to the left of the item.

   Fitbit deletes the food item.

Tracking Your Food Plan

The nice thing about having a food plan is that if you stick with it — that is, if you match your daily calorie deficit (give or take a few calories either way) — you *will* eventually reach your target weight. Nice. To help you get there, Fitbit offers tools for tracking both your daily calorie deficits and your overall weight loss.

Tracking your daily calorie deficit

You might think that you have to wait until the end of the day to see whether you met your target calorie deficit for the day. Not so! Fitbit not only enables you to monitor your net calories (that is, calories in minus calories out), but also slots your current net calories into one of three categories:

» **In Zone:** Your net calories are on pace to meet your daily calorie deficit target.

» **Under Target:** Your net calories are a bit low, meaning you're in danger of coming in too far under your calorie deficit target. That might sound like a good thing, but it's better to stick with your plan and keep your net calories in the In Zone category. When it comes to losing weight, patience is a virtue.

» **Over Target:** Your net calories are a bit high, meaning you might go too far over your calorie deficit target.

To see today's current values for calories in, calories out, how many calories you have left to reach your calorie deficit target, and your calorie category, use either of the following techniques:

» **Fitbit app:** In the Dashboard, click the Food Plan tile to open the Food screen, shown in Figure 10-8. The Cals In Vs Out graph shows your daily calories in (the left bar) and calories out (the right bar), with the calories-in bar color-coded according to your calorie category (green for In Zone, blue for Under Target, and red for Over Target). Below the graph, the Today section shows your current calorie numbers.

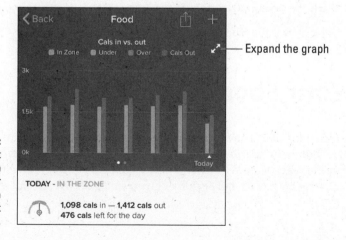

FIGURE 10-8: Click the Fitbit app's Food Plan tile to see your calorie graph and current calorie values.

» **Fitbit.com:** Log in to display the Dashboard, and then check out the Calories In vs Out tile, shown on the left in Figure 10-9, which displays calories in (left) versus calories out (right), plus a meter that displays your current calorie deficit category. The Food Plan tile, shown on the right in Figure 10-9, displays how many calories you have left to consume today. (Hover the mouse pointer over the Food Plan tile to see your current calories-in value and your total allowed calories.)

Calories In vs Out tile   Food Plan tile

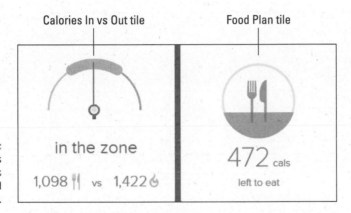

FIGURE 10-9:
Fitbit.com offers
Calories In vs
Out and Food
Plan tiles.

in the zone

1,098 🍴 vs 1,422 🔥

472 cals

left to eat

Tracking your overall weight loss

The point of creating a food plan, logging everything you eat, keeping a close eye on your daily calorie deficit, and pumping up your calories burned with regular exercise and activities is, of course, to lose pounds (or kilograms, as the case may be) and reach your target weight. For incentive or inspiration, use either of the following techniques to monitor your overall weight loss since you began your plan:

» **Fitbit app:** In the Dashboard, the Weight tile (see Figure 10-10, left) shows how many pounds you've lost (I hope), as well as a semicircle that shows how far along you are to your goal weight.

» **Fitbit.com:** Log in to display the Dashboard, and then examine the Weight tile (see Figure 10-10, right), which shows how many pounds you still have to lose to reach your goal weight, as well as a semicircle that shows how far along you are to your target. (Hover the mouse pointer over the Weight tile to see your current weight and your starting and target weight values.)

FIGURE 10-10:
The Fitbit app
shows how many
pounds you've
lost (left); Fitbit.
com shows how
many pounds you
have to lose.

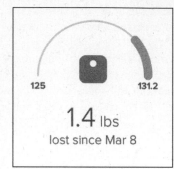

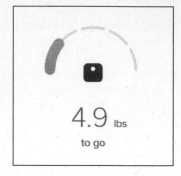

IN THIS CHAPTER

» Learning how to sit less and move more

» Getting yourself to exercise regularly

» Maintaining that ideal weight you worked so hard to achieve

» Setting up regular bedtimes and wake-up times

» Getting into the habit of drinking enough water

» Using deep breathing and meditation to calm yourself

Chapter **11**

Developing Healthier Habits

I f you want to feel good both mentally and physically, there's nothing like exercising, eating a nutritious meal, and getting a good night's sleep. The positive vibes you feel afterward are your body's way of saying "Thanks!" Wouldn't it be great to feel that good all (or at least most) of the time? That goal might sound like a pipe dream, but it's within reach for most people. The secret is taking those health-promoting exercises, meals, and sleeps and upgrading them from irregular happenings to full-blown habits. When good-for-you activities go from something you do once in a while or with a goal in mind (such as losing weight) to something you just do, period, ruddy-cheeked, endorphin-bathed health is sure to follow.

Yep, it does take a while to form the health habit, but fortunately you're not alone in your quest. Your Fitbit tracker is right there, by your side, ready to lend a helping hand. In this chapter, you explore the many ways that you can use your Fitbit device, app, and account to develop solid and long-lasting healthier habits for activity, eating, sleeping, reducing stress, and more.

Healthy Habit #1: Sitting Less and Moving More

Just last weekend, my local newspaper had a big article about how sitting too much not only leads to the usual problems of inactivity (cardiovascular disease, backaches, muscle atrophy, bone deterioration, and more) but also offsets the healthful properties of exercise. Which weekend was that? It doesn't matter because you can probably look in any newspaper or news website and see a similar story. Life has few certainties, but one is that sitting for long periods is really, really, *really* bad for you.

You learn everything you need to know to use your Fitbit to avoid over–sitting in Chapter 5. Here's a summary:

>> **Turn on Fitbit's Reminders to Move.** At ten minutes to the hour, Fitbit reminds you to get up and move if you haven't yet reached 250 steps for that hour. In the Fitbit app, click the Hourly Activity tile, click the Settings icon, labeled in Figure 11-1, and then click the Reminders to Move switch to on (green).

>> **Extend your Reminders to Move hours.** You can ask Fitbit to remind you to move at least 250 steps each hour for up to 14 consecutive hours. In the Fitbit app, click the Hourly Activity tile, click the Settings icon (gear), and then use the Start Time and End Time settings to specify when Reminders to Move are in force.

>> **Look for times when you regularly don't move.** We all have movement blind spots: hours during the day when we regularly don't reach those 250 steps. Remember that it takes only a few minutes of walking to reach 250 steps, so there's no excuse for not reaching that modest goal. To look for your own blind spots, click the Fitbit app's Hourly Activity tile, and then examine the Hours with 250+ Steps graph, shown in Figure 11-1. The red dots represent hours in which you reached the 250-step goal. Examine the graph vertically to look for hours that have few or no dots. Those are your blind spots.

>> **Keep an eye on your longest stationary period.** You should not only move regularly — ideally, every half hour or so — but also make sure that the longest period you sit during the day is less than two hours and ideally less than one hour. Fitbit tracks both the longest period each day that you don't move and your 30-day average longest stationary period. To see these metrics, click the Fitbit app's Hourly Activity tile, swipe left on the Hours with 250+ Steps graph (in Windows 10, click the > icon). Fitbit displays the Longest Stationary Period graph, shown in Figure 11-2. You see your longest non-movement time for the past week, as well as a vertical bar that shows your 30-day average stationary time.

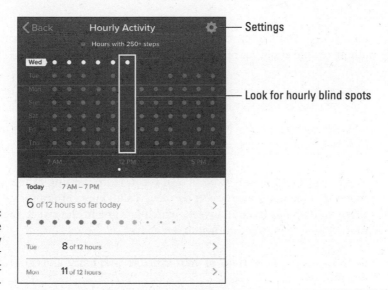

Settings —

Look for hourly blind spots —

FIGURE 11-1:
Examine the graph vertically to find your movement blind spots.

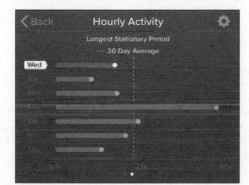

FIGURE 11-2:
Try to get your average longest stationary period below two hours.

Healthy Habit #2: Exercising Regularly

Going out for a brisk walk, run, or bike ride is a great way to do something good for your body. If you do these and similar exercises once in a while, you'll feel good for a day, but if you exercise regularly, you'll feel good pretty much all the time. Okay, fine, but what do I mean by *regularly*? According to the document *Physical Activity Guidelines for Americans* published by the U.S. Department of Health and Human Services (and echoed by just about every health expert in the world), adults should shoot for one of the following:

>> Between 150 minutes (two and a half hours) and 300 minutes (five hours) of moderate intensity exercise per week.

>> Between 75 minutes (one and a quarter hours) and 150 minutes (two and a half hours) of vigorous intensity exercise per week.

Most health and fitness experts also recommend getting at least 30 minutes of moderate-intensity exercise every day. That daily minimum gets you at least three and a half hours in a week, which is right in the sweet spot of the weekly moderate-intensity recommendation above.

So, how do you keep track of your exercise frequency and duration? Fitbit gives you four ways:

>> **Set an exercise goal:** This goal refers to the number of days per week that you exercise. In the Fitbit app, click Dashboard ⇨ Account, click Exercise, click the goal value, and then select the number of days you want to shoot for. That value might be as little as three or four days when you're just starting out, but eventually you'll want to bump it up to six or, ideally, seven days.

>> **Track your weekly exercise minutes:** In the Fitbit app, click the Weekly Exercise tile to open the Exercise screen, shown in Figure 11-3. The top of the screen shows you the number of days of exercise you've completed so far, but it also includes a This Week value, which displays your total exercise time so far this week.

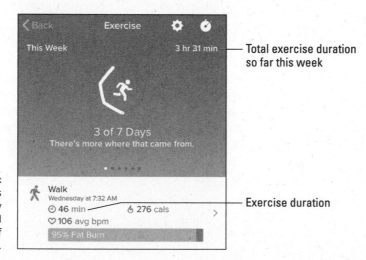

FIGURE 11-3:
Fitbit displays your total weekly exercise time and the duration of each exercise.

Total exercise duration so far this week

Exercise duration

>> **Track the duration of each exercise:** In the Fitbit app, click the Weekly Exercise tile to open the Exercise screen. Below the graph, you see an entry for each exercise session, which includes the duration of the exercise, as labeled in Figure 11-3.

>> **Track your daily exercise duration:** In the Fitbit app, click the Weekly Exercise tile to open the Exercise screen. Then swipe left (in the Windows 10 app, click the > icon) twice to display the Duration (Minutes) graph, shown in Figure 11-4. This graph tells you the number of minutes of exercise you've done each day for the past month.

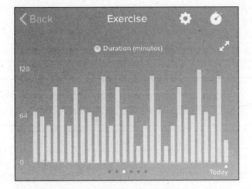

FIGURE 11-4:
Use the Duration (Minutes) graph to track your daily exercise duration.

Healthy Habit #3: Maintaining Your Ideal Weight

In Chapter 10, I show you how to use Fitbit and your Fitbit account to help you lose weight by setting a goal weight and then creating a food plan with a specified calorie deficit. After you get to your target weight (congratulations, by the way!), your new goal should be to maintain that weight, which means balancing the calories you consume with the calories you burn. In other words, you want to run a calorie deficit of zero (give or take a few calories).

To help keep your current weight, change your weight goal from losing weight to maintaining weight. Here are the steps to follow:

1. **In the Fitbit app, click Dashboard ⇨ Account.**

2. **In the Goals section, click Nutrition & Body.**

3. **In Android or iOS, click Goal Weight. In Windows 10, click the Goal Weight text box, enter your current weight, and then skip the rest of these steps.**

   Fitbit asks whether you want to lose, gain, or maintain weight.

4. **Click Maintain.**

   Fitbit asks if you have a body fat percentage goal.

5. **Click Skip.**

   Fitbit saves your goal.

Healthy Habit #4: Setting Up a Sleep Schedule

In Chapter 6, I explain Fitbit's sleep metrics, including time asleep and the sleep stages (light, deep, REM, and awake). However, I didn't cover one metric: sleep schedule. Your sleep schedule is perhaps the most straightforward of the sleep metrics: It's the time you go to bed (that is, when you turn out the light) and the time you get out of bed in the morning. However, don't let that simplicity fool you, because your sleep schedule is an important part of your overall sleep hygiene. Specifically, consistent bedtimes and wake-up times have been shown to promote good sleep habits and better sleep quality overall.

Here are the steps to follow to set up a sleep schedule:

1. **In the Fitbit app. click Dashboard ⇨ Account.**

2. **In the Goals section, click Sleep.**

   The Sleep Goals screen appears.

3. **Click the Bedtime setting.**

   If you've been tracking your sleep, Fitbit displays your average time in bed, as shown in Figure 11-5. Fitbit asks if this is enough rest for you.

WARNING

Fitbit describes the displayed time as *your average sleep,* but that's not accurate because you most likely spent some of that time awake. The displayed value is really the amount of time you spent in bed. The problem is that, after you go through the sleep schedule process outlined in these steps, Fitbit takes this time-in-bed value (or the value you specify in Step 4) and sets it as your new time asleep goal! Boo, Fitbit! This confusion means you'll probably have to adjust your time asleep goal when you finish setting up your sleep schedule.

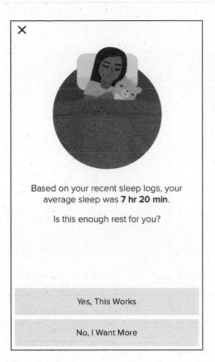

FIGURE 11-5:
Fitbit displays
your average
time in bed.

Based on your recent sleep logs, your average sleep was **7 hr 20 min**.

Is this enough rest for you?

Yes, This Works

No, I Want More

4. **Click one of the displayed options:**

- **Yes, This Works:** You feel like you're getting a good night's sleep. Fitbit rounds off the time in bed to the nearest 15 minutes and asks if you want to set this time as your goal.

- **No, I Want More:** You don't think you're getting enough rest. Fitbit adds a half hour or so to the time in bed, rounded to the nearest 15 minutes, and asks if you want to set this time as your goal, as shown in Figure 11-6.

5. **Click one of the displayed options:**

- **Make This My Goal:** Accept Fitbit's suggested total time in bed.

- **Set Different Goal:** Specify the hours and minutes you want for your time in bed goal, and then click Save.

Fitbit tells you your goal is set and that it's now ready to set your sleep schedule.

6. **Click Next.**

Fitbit shows your average wake-up time, as shown in Figure 11-7.

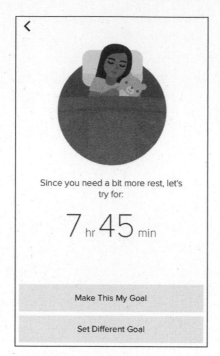

FIGURE 11-6:
Fitbit displays
your new time
in bed goal.

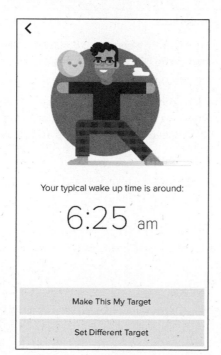

FIGURE 11-7:
Fitbit suggests a
wake-up time.

7. **Click one of the displayed options:**

- **Make This My Target:** Accept Fitbit's suggested wake-up time.

- **Set Different Target:** Specify the time you want to wake up, and then click Save.

Fitbit asks if you want to set a silent alarm on your tracker to wake you at the time you specified in Step 7.

8. **Click one of the displayed options:**

- **Set Silent Alarm:** Set the wake-up alarm, and then click Next when Fitbit tells you the alarm will be added to your tracker the next time you sync.

- **Not Right Now:** Skip the alarm.

Fitbit suggests a bedtime based on your wake-up time, time in bed, and how long it typically takes you to fall asleep, as shown in Figure 11-8.

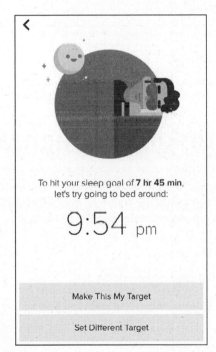

FIGURE 11-8:
Fitbit suggests
a bedtime.

9. **Click one of the displayed options:**

- **Make This My Target:** Accept Fitbit's suggested bedtime.

- **Set Different Target:** Specify the time you want to go to bed, and then click Save.

Fitbit asks if you want to set a bedtime reminder, which is a notification that appears on your tracker (and your smartphone) a half hour before it's time to hit the hay. By default, Fitbit displays these reminders only Sunday through Thursday.

10. **Click one of the displayed options:**

- **Yes, Remind Me:** Accept Fitbit's suggested reminder time and the default reminder days.

- **Customize My Reminder:** Specify the time you want to be reminded as well as which days you see the reminders, and then click Save.

- **Skip:** Bypass the bedtime reminders.

Fitbit lets you know that your sleep schedule is ready to go.

11. **Click All Done.**

Fitbit configures your tracker as needed the next time you sync.

Healthy Habit #5: Drinking Enough Water

One of the often overlooked aspects of good health is drinking enough water every day. Having an adequate daily intake of water is associated with a long list of your-body-will-thank-you outcomes, including the following:

>> Regulating your internal temperature

>> Keeping your joints lubricated and cushioned

>> Protecting tissues

>> Promoting waste removal, especially through sweating and urination

>> Helping you lose weight

>> Keeping your energy levels high throughout the day

>> Helping with health problems such as dry skin, hand and foot cramps, constipation, acne, and kidney stones

Okay, so when I write about drinking enough water every day, what do I mean by *enough*? I just *knew* you were going to ask that!

Whenever the conversation turns to making sure we drink enough water during the day — you *do* have these water-intake conversations, don't you? — someone always trots out the so-called 8x8 rule: Drink an eight-ounce glass of water at least eight times a day. The 8x8 rule looks like a good rule, doesn't it? It's pithy and it's easy to understand, so that's the end of the conversation, right?

Actually, no, it's not. The problem, you see, is that 8x8 has no scientific basis! No evidence supports drinking that amount of water each day. 8x8 is just an arbitrary amount of water and should really be renamed to 0x0 because it's supported by zero evidence and zero justification.

So, again, how much water is enough? First, understand that you get plenty of water from the foods you eat, particularly if you eat healthy foods such as fruit and vegetables. (And most meats, fish, and eggs are also great sources of water.)

TIP

Many foods and liquids are around 90 percent water, which means they can contribute significantly to your daily water intake. Examples of water-abundant items include bell peppers, broth, cantaloupe, cauliflower, cucumber, grapefruit, lettuce, oranges, peaches, soup (usually), skim milk, strawberries, tomatoes, watermelon, and zucchini.

Second, know that you also get loads of water from beverages such as coffee and tea. Yes, coffee and tea are diuretic (meaning they tend to make you urinate), but the water you lose is much less than the water you take in, so the net benefit, water-wise, is positive.

Third, your body has an excellent and pretty much foolproof internal mechanism for maintaining the correct amount of water (around 60 percent of body weight for most folks). The long and the short of the internal water-maintenance regulator is this:

> If your body detects that you're running low on water, it makes you thirsty.

Yep, that's it. As long as you drink some water whenever you're thirsty, you don't have to give your water needs much thought. Well, there are some important exceptions to this let-your-body-regulate-your-water idea:

>> When you exercise, drink lots of water (that is, don't wait until you're thirsty).

>> If you live in a dry climate or if it's hot outside, drink water regularly.

>> If you're breastfeeding, drink extra water.

>> If you have a medical problem that causes vomiting or diarrhea, drink lots of water to make up for what you're losing.

Otherwise, if you're healthy and none of the preceding exceptions apply to you, you'll be fine as long as you listen to your body telling you when it's time to drink water. Ah, but the key phrase here is *as long as you listen to your body*, which, alas, is not the case for many of us. You get busy with work or play or social media, and before you know it, you've gone the entire day without drinking any water. Your body has probably been lighting up the "Thirsty" light for a while now (when things get bad your body might also flash the "Hungry" light in a desperate bid for *any* source of water).

If you regularly miss your body's thirst cues, it's time to get your Fitbit on the job to remind you to drink water during the day. That reminder comes in the form of a water goal, which is a specified number of ounces (or milliliters) you want to consume throughout the day.

Calculating a water goal

What should you water goal be? That depends on your health, what you eat, how much you exercise, and your local climate. I suggest spending a few days or a week monitoring your thirst and drinking some water (try 8 ounces or 250 milliliters) whenever thirst arises. Multiply the average number of times per day that you feel thirsty during this trial period by the number of ounces or milliliters you drink each time. The result should be a good start for your water goal.

Set a water goal by using the Fitbit app

Here are the steps to follow to set your daily water goal by using the Fitbit app:

1. **Click Dashboard ⇨ Account.**

2. **In the Goals section, click Nutrition & Body.**

3. **Under Nutrition, click the Water value and then enter the number of ounces or milliliters (depending on your liquid unit of choice).**

4. **Click the Back icon (<).**

    The app syncs the new goal to your Fitbit.

Set a water goal by using Fitbit.com

Follow these steps online to set your daily water goal by using Fitbit.com:

1. Surf over to www.fitbit.com and log in to your account to display the Dashboard.

2. Hover the mouse pointer over the Water tile, and then click the Settings icon (the gear) that appears below the tile.

3. In the Daily Goal box, enter the number of ounces or milliliters.

4. Click Done.

Fitbit saves the new goal and adds it to your Fitbit the next time you sync.

Logging your water intake

To know how much water you're consuming each day and how close that consumption is getting you to your daily water goal, you need to log your water intake by using one of the following methods:

TIP

>> **Ionic or Versa watch:** From the clock, swipe up from the bottom of the screen to open the Today app, and then swipe up until you see the Water metric. Tap Water, tap the amount of water you consumed, and then tap the check mark.

If you don't see the Water metric in the Today app, scroll to the bottom of the Today app, tap Settings, and then tap to select the Water check box. If the Water check box is disabled, tap to deselect one of the other core stats, and then tap to select Water.

>> **Fitbit app:** In the Dashboard, tap the Log icon (+) and then tap Log Water. In the Add Water Log screen (see Figure 11-9), either type the amount of water you drank or click one of the icons in the Quick Add section.

>> **Fitbit.com:** After logging in, click Log in the main navigation bar and then click the Food tab, or surf directly to www.fitbit.com/foods/log. Near the bottom of the page, type the amount of water you consumed, click a unit, and then click Log It.

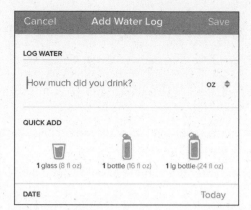

FIGURE 11-9:
Use the Fitbit
app's Add Water
Log screen to log
your water
consumption.

Tracking your water intake

To keep an eye on your daily water consumption, use any of the following techniques:

» **Ionic or Versa watch:** From the clock, swipe up from the bottom of the screen to open the Today app, and then swipe up until you see the Water metric.

» **Fitbit app:** Open the Dashboard and examine the Water tile, shown in Figure 11-10). You can also click the Water tile to see your historical data for water consumption.

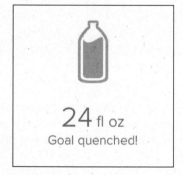

FIGURE 11-10:
The Fitbit app's
Water tile tracks
today's water
consumption.

» **Fitbit.com:** Log in to display the Dashboard, and then examine the Water tile. You can also hover the mouse pointer over the Water tile and then click Quick View to see you water drinking history.

Healthy Habit #6: Reducing Stress

Telling someone your life is stressful is a dangerous move because the other person will almost certainly respond with multiple tales of woe about how stressful his or her life is, which only adds to your own stress. We're all stressed out these days, but you'll be happy to hear that your Fitbit can help here, too. In fact, I've already talked about quite a few ways that your Fitbit can help you de-stress:

>> Getting plenty of activity and exercise is the ideal stress-buster.

>> Reaching your ideal weight gives you one less thing to fret about during your day.

>> Getting enough sleep every night is one of the best ways to get a calm, refreshed start to the day and to keep that calm mood going for most of the day.

>> Eating healthy foods and drinking enough water are surefire ways to boost your energy and help keep the stress demons at bay.

Unfortunately, these techniques aren't enough to guarantee a stress-free day, especially when a deadline looms, your coworkers are particularly crazy, or your boss asks for the impossible yet again. When the stress becomes just about intolerable, try to get away for five or ten minutes (or more, if you can). Find a comfortable place to sit, and then de-stress using one of the following apps on your Fitbit:

>> **Relax:** This app offers guided deep-breathing sessions. After first sensing your breathing, the app uses screen imagery and tracker vibrations to prompt you to inhale deeply and slowly and then exhale just as slowly. The default session is two minutes, but you can tap the Settings icon (gear) to change the duration.

>> **Timer:** If you prefer more traditional meditation, use the Timer app's Countdown timer feature. Set the timer to however long you want to meditate and then tap the Start button. If you're new to meditation, close your eyes (or keep them open; your choice), and then breath normally. Find the place where you most readily feel your breath (the nostrils, chest, or stomach), and direct your attention to that area. When you notice that your mind has wandered (and it *will* wander), gently and non-judgmentally direct your attention back to the breath. Repeat until your tracker vibrates to signal the end of the session.

4

The Part of Tens

Chapter **12**

Ten Troubleshooting Techniques

Fitbits look like simple devices from the outside, but even the least complicated Fitbits — such as the Ace and Inspire — have sophisticated innards bristling with sensors, storage, and other electronic trinkets and gewgaws. Surprisingly, all this internal gimcrackery has no moving parts! Nothing spins or whirls or flips, which is great news because it's less likely that something will break, even if you drop your Fitbit. Chances are good that you'll go your entire Fitbit career without having any problems.

Notice I wrote *chances are good*, not *chances are 100 percent*. I'm hedging my bets here because your Fitbit is still digital technology — and have you ever used a digital device or software that worked flawlessly all the time? I thought not. So, yep, it's entirely possible that one day your Fitbit will start doing weird things or even stop working. In this chapter, you investigate the most common problems related to Fitbit hardware and software, and learn many useful solutions.

General Troubleshooting Techniques

TIP

Before getting to the specific problems and their solutions, I want to take you through a few basic troubleshooting steps. Many problems can be solved by doing the following three things (each of which I explain in more detail in the sections that follow):

>> Restart your Fitbit.

>> Update your Fitbit's software.

>> Reset your Fitbit to its factory default settings.

REMEMBER

Try restarting your Fitbit to see if it solves your problem. If not, move on to updating the software (assuming an update is available) and see if that helps. If there's still no joy, only then should you try resetting your Fitbit to its factory default settings.

Restarting your Fitbit

If your Fitbit is having trouble connecting to Wi-Fi, syncing, or doing any of its normal duties, by far the most common solution is to restart the device. By rebooting the device, you reload the system, which is often enough to solve many problems.

REMEMBER

When you restart your Fitbit, you don't lose any stored data, your settings are preserved, and you keep connections such as Wi-Fi networks and Bluetooth devices.

How you restart depends on which Fitbit you have:

>> **Ace, Alta, or Alta HR:** Clip your charging cable to your Fitbit and plug the other end of the cable into a USB port. On the USB end of the cable, locate the small button and press it three times within eight seconds, pausing briefly between each press.

>> **Aria 2:** On the bottom of the Aria, remove the battery cover, remove the batteries, wait ten seconds, reinsert the batteries, and then replace the battery cover.

>> **Charge 3:** If your device interface still works, open the Settings app and tap Reboot Device. If your device is locked up, attach one end of your charging cable to the Fitbit and the other to a USB port, and then press and hold down the device's button (labeled in Chapter 3) for eight seconds.

- » **Flex 2:** Remove the Flex 2 from its wristband, clip your charging cable to your Fitbit, and plug the other end of the cable into a USB port. Find the small button on the USB end of the cable and press the button three times within five seconds, pausing briefly between each press.

- » **Ionic or Versa:** Press and hold down the Back and Bottom buttons (labeled in Chapter 3) until you see the Fitbit logo.

- » **Inspire or Inspire HR:** Press and hold down the device button for five seconds.

- » **Zip:** Use the battery door tool to open the battery door. Then remove the battery, wait impatiently for ten seconds, reinsert the battery (making sure the side with the + icon is facing you), and then close the battery door.

Updating your Fitbit

Your Fitbit uses internal software — often called *firmware* — to perform all sorts of tasks, including operating the sensors, storing data, keeping time, and running apps. If your Fitbit is acting wonky and restarting the device doesn't help, you can often de-wonkify the device by updating the Fitbit system software. Sometimes installing a fresh version of the software is all you need to make your problem go away. In other cases, updating the software may fix a software glitch that was causing your problem.

Happily, all Fitbits update their software automatically. When an update is available, the Fitbit app displays a notification similar to the one shown in Figure 12-1. Tap the Update icon (downward-pointing arrow) to perform the update.

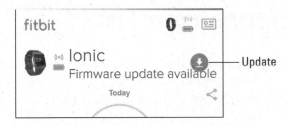

FIGURE 12-1:
When a Fitbit firmware update is available, you see a notification similar to this.

Resetting your Fitbit

If your problem is particularly ornery, restarting or updating the device won't solve it. In that case, you need to take the drastic step of a *factory reset*, which means resetting your Fitbit to its original factory settings. I describe the factory reset as *drastic* because it means you lose your data and settings and you have to go through the setup process again. Ouch. Therefore, only head down reset road if restarting and updating your device don't solve the problem.

However, not all Fitbits come with a factory reset option. Specifically, there's no reset for you if you own any of the following models:

>> **Ace**

>> **Alta**

>> **Alta HR**

>> **Flex 2**

>> **Inspire**

>> **Inspire HR**

>> **Zip**

For all the rest, how you perform the reset depends on your device:

>> **Aria 2:** On the bottom of the Aria, remove the battery cover, remove the batteries, and then press and hold down the button just above the battery slots. While holding down the button for at least ten seconds, reinsert the batteries. When you're finished, replace the battery cover.

>> **Charge 3:** Open the Settings app and then tap About ⇨ Clear User Data.

>> **Ionic or Versa:** Open the Settings app and then tap About ⇨ Factory Reset.

You Can't Configure Your Fitbit

As I describe in Chapter 3, you use the Fitbit app to connect with and configure your Fitbit device. If you can't install the app, connect to your device, or run the configuration, here are some troubleshooting ideas to try:

>> If you're trying to configure a Fitbit Ace, remember that the Ace device requires special setup steps, as I describe in Chapter 4.

>> Make sure your phone, tablet, or Windows 10 version is compatible with the Fitbit app (see Chapter 3).

>> Your Fitbit might be having trouble syncing with your phone, tablet, or PC, so try out the solutions in this chapter's "Your Fitbit Won't Sync" section.

>> Make sure your phone, tablet, or PC is running the latest version of its operating system:

- *Android:* Tap Settings ➪ Software Update ➪ Download Updates Manually.

- *iOS:* Tap Settings ➪ General ➪ Software Update.

- *Windows 10:* Click Start ➪ Settings ➪ Update & Security, make sure the Windows Update tab is displayed, and then click Check for Updates.

>> Reboot your Fitbit as I described earlier in the "Restarting your Fitbit" section.

>> Reboot the phone, tablet, or PC that's running the Fitbit app.

>> Remove your Fitbit device (and any other Fitbit devices you've added) from the Fitbit app and then try adding your Fitbit device again.

>> Uninstall and then reinstall the Fitbit app.

You Can't Update Your Fitbit

Earlier in this chapter I talk briefly about updating your Fitbit and mention that it was usually a blissfully uneventful procedure. Usually, but unfortunately not always. Every once in a while, you might find that a firmware update fails to start, fails to finish, or goes south on you in some other way. If updates aren't happening for you, here, in order, are some troubleshooting steps to try:

>> Restart your tracker as I describe previously in the "Restarting your Fitbit" section, and then try updating again.

>> Restart the phone, tablet, or PC that has the Fitbit app installed, and then try the update once more.

>> Install the Fitbit app on a different phone, tablet, or PC, configure your Fitbit account on that device, set up your Fitbit, and then try updating.

If you have an Ionic or Versa watch, here are some extra troubleshooting ideas to consider:

>> Make sure your watch is either charging or has a battery charge of at least 40 percent.

>> If you're updating over Wi-Fi, try the troubleshooting steps that I outline later in the "Your Fitbit Watch Can't Connect to Wi-Fi" section.

>> If you're updating over Bluetooth, try the Bluetooth-related troubleshooting steps that appear later in the "Your Fitbit Won't Sync" section.

Your Fitbit Won't Sync

When you open the Fitbit app, as long as your Fitbit device is nearby, the device should sync its data with the app (and vice versa). Ah, but that *should* is no consolation when your Fitbit is bursting with useful data but you can't get the Fitbit app to sync.

When your tracker refuses to sync, here are a few troubleshooting techniques to run through (in the order listed):

>> Check that your Fitbit is either charging or its battery life isn't nearly done (that is, under 10 percent).

>> Make sure your phone, tablet, or PC has Bluetooth turned on:

- *Android:* Tap Settings ⇨ Connections, and then tap the Bluetooth switch to On.

- *iOS:* Tap Settings ⇨ Bluetooth, and then tap the Bluetooth switch to on (green).

- *Windows 10:* Click Start ⇨ Settings ⇨ Devices, make sure the Bluetooth and Other Devices tab is displayed, and then click the Bluetooth switch to On.

>> Using the appropriate method in the preceding bullet, turn or your phone, tablet, or PC Bluetooth setting, and then turn it back on again.

>> Remove the Fitbit from the list of paired Bluetooth devices on your phone, tablet, or PC, as described next, remove the device from the Fitbit app, and then set up the device again in the Fitbit app:

- *Android:* Tap Settings ⇨ Connections ⇨ Bluetooth, tap the Settings icon (gear) to the right of your Fitbit device, and then tap Unpair.

- *iOS:* Tap Settings ⇨ Bluetooth, tap the Info icon (i), and then tap Forget This Device.

- *Windows 10:* Click Start ⇨ Settings ⇨ Devices, make sure the Bluetooth and Other Devices tab is displayed, click your Fitbit, and then click Remove Device.

>> If you're syncing multiple Fitbits, make sure the other Fitbit devices aren't nearby.

>> Make sure your phone, tablet, or Windows 10 version is compatible with the Fitbit app (see Chapter 3).

>> Make sure you're using the latest version of the Fitbit app.

>> Make sure your phone, tablet, or PC is running the latest version of its operating system:

- *Android:* Tap Settings ⇨ Software Update ⇨ Download Updates Manually.

- *iOS:* Tap Settings ⇨ General ⇨ Software Update.

- *Windows 10:* Click Start ⇨ Settings ⇨ Update & Security, make sure the Windows Update tab is displayed, and then click Check for Updates.

>> Restart the Fitbit device as I described previously in the "Restarting your Fitbit" section.

>> Reboot the phone, tablet, or PC that's running the Fitbit app.

>> Remove your Fitbit device (and any other Fitbit devices you've added) from the Fitbit app and then try adding your Fitbit device again.

>> Uninstall and then reinstall the Fitbit app.

>> Install the Fitbit app on a different phone, tablet, or PC. Configure your Fitbit account on that device, set up your Fitbit, and then try syncing.

Your Fitbit Isn't Receiving Notifications

Having your smartphone notifications appear on your Fitbit is a nice bonus feature because it enables you to quickly check an incoming notification without having to pull out your phone. That convenience is lost if your Fitbit no longer displays those notifications, however. Cue the hair pulling and gnashing of teeth.

Let go of that hair! Here are some troubleshooting techniques to try, instead:

>> Make sure your Fitbit is within range (about 30 feet) of your smartphone.

>> Check that your smartphone is itself displaying notifications. If, for example, your smartphone is in Do Not Disturb mode (or a similar mode, depending on your device), where it temporarily shuts off notifications, you won't see any notifications on your Fitbit.

>> Make sure your Fitbit device is configured to receive notifications. For the Charge 3, Ionic, or Versa, press and hold down the device's Back button to display the Quick Settings, and then tap the Notifications setting to On.

» If you're not receiving certain types of notification, use the Fitbit app to click Dashboard ⇨ Account. Click your Fitbit device, click Notifications, and then make sure the switch is On for the notification type you're missing.

» Make sure your phone, tablet, or PC has Bluetooth turned on:

- *Android:* Tap Settings ⇨ Connections, and then tap the Bluetooth switch to On.

- *iOS:* Tap Settings ⇨ Bluetooth, and then tap the Bluetooth switch to on (green).

- *Windows 10:* Click Start ⇨ Settings ⇨ Devices, make sure the Bluetooth and Other Devices tab is displayed, and then click the Bluetooth switch to On.

» Using the appropriate method in the preceding bullet, turn off your phone, tablet, or PC Bluetooth setting, and then turn it back on again.

» Restart the Fitbit device as I describe previously in the "Restarting your Fitbit" section.

» Remove your Fitbit device (and any other Fitbit devices you've added) from the Fitbit app and then try adding your Fitbit device again.

You're Having Fitbit Battery Troubles

All Fitbits run on battery power, so it can really kill your tracking buzz to have battery woes, which means either that your Fitbit is going through juice annoyingly fast or you can't charge your Fitbit battery.

Checking the Fitbit battery level

First, here are the various ways you can check your Fitbit's current battery level:

» **Ace, Alta, or Alta HR:** Wake the device and then tap the screen until you see the battery level icon.

» **Charge 3:** From the clock, swipe up once.

» **Inspire or Inspire HR:** Press the device button for a few seconds.

» **Ionic or Versa:** From the clock, swipe up from the bottom of the screen to display the Today app, which shows the current battery level in the upper-left corner, as shown in Figure 12-2.

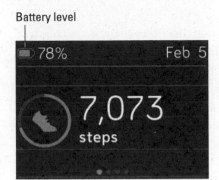

Battery level

FIGURE 12-2:
The battery level
on an Ionic or
Versa watch.

>> **Fitbit app:** An icon for your Fitbit device appears at the top of the Dashboard screen and includes a battery level icon, as shown in Figure 12-3. If you have multiple connected Fitbits, click Dashboard ⇨ Account. The Account screen displays your connected Fitbit devices, each of which includes a battery icon.

>> **Fitbit.com:** Log in to open the Dashboard and then click View Settings. The page that appears shows each Fitbit device and its current battery level.

Battery level

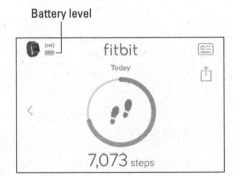

FIGURE 12-3:
The battery level
in the Fitbit app.

TIP

You can configure your Fitbit account to receive an email notification when you Fitbit battery hits 25 percent. In the Fitbit app, click Dashboard, then Account, then Notifications. Click the Low Battery switch to On.

Your Fitbit's battery life is too short

How much battery life you get from your Fitbit depends on many factors, includ-ing the apps you use and the settings you've chosen. If you're getting battery life that's significantly shorter than the times I outline in Chapter 2, you should consider one or more of the following solutions:

>> Turn off Quick View, which is the feature that wakes the Fitbit when you turn your wrist towards you. How you turn off Quick View depends on the device:

- *Charge 3, Ionic, or Versa:* Press and hold down the Back button to open the Quick Settings, and then tap the Screen Wake setting to Off.

- *All other Fitbits:* In the Fitbit app, click Dashboard ⇨ Account, and then click the Quick View switch to Off.

>> Turn off notifications if you're receiving lots of them.

>> Reduce the number of hourly activity reminders (that is, the reminders that appear when you haven't hit 250 steps in the hour). The best way to prevent these reminders is to get in your 250 steps each hour. You can also reduce the number of hours that you want your Fitbit to remind you to move (see Chapter 5).

>> Reduce the number of silent alarms you've set up.

>> Turn off heart rate monitoring if you don't use it.

>> Don't play media or use apps that keep your screen activated.

>> With an Ionic or Versa, don't extend the minimum time that the display stays on when you wake the device. Open Settings and then use the Display Awake setting to choose a short duration, such as 10 seconds.

>> Only charge your Fitbit in moderate temperatures.

Your Fitbit isn't charging

If your Fitbit won't charge at all, here are some typical problems and troubleshooting ideas to work through:

>> **Your Fitbit is plugged into a USB hub or wall charger that doesn't supply power.** Try plugging the Fitbit into a USB device or charger that does supply AC power.

>> **The Fitbit charging cable isn't connected securely to the Fitbit.** Double-check the connection.

>> **Your Fitbit's charging contacts or the pins on the charging cable are dirty or are surrounded by dust or debris.** Try blowing on the contacts and pins to clear away any dust or debris. If your Fitbit still won't charge, wet a cotton swab with a small amount of rubbing alcohol and then use the swab to clean the contacts and pins. Dry the contacts and pins before attempting to charge the Fitbit.

If none of the above work for you, restart your Fitbit, as I described earlier in the "Restarting your Fitbit" section.

>> **Your USB hub or wall charger is defective.** Try a different USB device.

>> **Your Fitbit is wet.** Try drying the Fitbit using the instructions I provide later in the "Your Fitbit Device Was Submerged in Water" section.

Your Fitbit Displays the Wrong Time

If your Fitbit is showing the wrong time, you can try two things right away: sync your Fitbit and change the time zone.

Your Fitbit might be temporarily time-deranged because of a recent time change (such as going into or out of Daylight Savings Time). Syncing your tracker with the Fitbit app should solve the problem.

If you travel into a different time zone, the Fitbit app should detect the new time zone based on your smartphone's updated location info. The automatic time zone change might not happen if you haven't configured the Fitbit app to set the time zone automatically (that is, based on your location) or if the Fitbit app can't access or determine your location. If you're in a new time zone and your Fitbit isn't displaying the correct local time, follow these steps to fix the problem:

1. **In the Fitbit app, click Dashboard ⇨ Account.**

2. **Click Advanced Settings.**

3. **(Windows 10 only) Click Time Zone.**

4. **Enable the Fitbit app to automatically set the time zone:**

   - *Android:* Tap the Automatic Time Zone switch to on (blue).

   - *iOS:* Tap the Set Automatically switch to on (green).

   - *Windows 10:* Tap the Auto switch to on (green).

5. **Sync your Fitbit and then check to see if the correct local time is displayed on the tracker.**

   If the correct local time is now displayed, say "Woo hoo!" and skip the rest of these steps, Otherwise, say "Boo hoo!", repeat Steps 1 through 3, and then continue with Step 6.

6. **Prevent the Fitbit app from automatically setting the time zone:**

   - *Android:* Tap the Automatic Time Zone switch to Off.

   - *iOS:* Tap the Set Automatically switch to Off.

   - *Windows 10:* Tap the Auto switch to Off and skip to Step 8.

7. **Tap Select Time Zone (Android) or Time Zone (iOS).**

8. **Select the time zone you're now in.**

9. **Sync your Fitbit.**

   Your Fitbit should now show the correct local time.

Your Fitbit Can't Connect to Wi-Fi

Wireless networking adds a new set of potential snags to your troubleshooting chores because of problems such as interference and device ranges. Here's a list of a few troubleshooting items that you should check to solve any wireless connectivity problems you're having with your Fitbit watch or Aria 2 scale:

>> **Restart your device(s).** Most Wi-Fi devices these days are all-in-one gadgets that combine both a Wi-Fi router and a modem for Internet access. If that's what you have, turn off the Wi-Fi device, wait a bit, turn the device back on, and then wait for the device to connect to your Internet provider. Restart your Fitbit as I describe earlier in the "Restarting your Fitbit" section.

Otherwise, if you have a separate router and modem, do the following tasks, in order:

1. **Turn off your modem.**

2. **Turn off your Wi-Fi router.**

3. **After a few seconds, turn the modem back on and wait until the modem reconnects to the Internet, which may take a few minutes.**

4. **Turn on your Wi-Fi router.**

5. **Restart your Fitbit as I describe earlier in the "Restarting your Fitbit" section.**

>> **Look for interference.** Devices such as baby monitors and cordless phones that use the 2.4 GHz radio frequency (RF) band can play havoc with wireless signals. Try either moving or turning off such devices if they're near your Fitbit or Wi-Fi device.

WARNING

Keep your Fitbit and Wi-Fi router well away from microwave ovens, which can jam wireless signals.

» **Check your range.** Your Fitbit may be too far away from the Wi-Fi router. You usually can't get much farther than about 230 feet away from most modern Wi-Fi devices before the signal begins to degrade (the range drops to about 115 feet for older Wi-Fi devices). Either move the Fitbit closer to the Wi-Fi router or turn on the router's range booster if it has one. You could also install a wireless range extender.

» **Check your password.** Make sure you're using the correct password to access your Wi-Fi network. It's also possible that your Wi-Fi device requires both Wi-Fi Protected Access (WPA) and Wi-Fi Protected Access II (WPA2) for extra security. Fitbit can deal with only one of these security types at a time, so if possible, configure your Wi-Fi device to use only WPA or WPA2. See your Wi-Fi device documentation to find out how to configure the device's security settings.

» **Update the wireless router firmware**. The wireless router firmware is the internal program that the router uses to perform its various chores. Wireless router manufacturers frequently update their firmware to fix bugs, so you should see whether an updated version of the firmware is available. Check your device documentation to find out how firmware updating works.

» **Update and optionally reset your Fitbit.** Make sure your Fitbit is up to date (see "Updating your Fitbit," previously in this chapter) and, if you still can't connect to Wi-Fi, reset your Fitbit (see "Resetting your Fitbit," earlier).

» **Reset the Wi-Fi device.** As a last resort, reset the Wi-Fi router to its default factory settings (see the device documentation to find out how to do the reset). Note that if you reset the router, you need to set up your network again from scratch.

Your Fitbit Device Can't Access GPS

Having access to a GPS signal makes your exercise tracking better because it enables you to see real-time pace and distance during the workout, gives you a final distance that's more accurate than calculating distance based on your stride length, and lets you view the route you took. GPS is a welcome addition to your tracking toolkit, but you lose the GPS advantage when your device can't access a GPS signal. How you resolve the problem depends on the Fitbit device you're using.

Troubleshooting GPS with a Charge 3 or Versa

If you have a Charge 3 wristband or Versa watch, those devices piggyback on your smartphone's GPS signal. Here are a few troubleshooting techniques to try if your Fitbit can't access GPS:

>> It can take a while for your Fitbit to establish a connection to the smartphone's GPS signal, so wait for a minute or two before deciding to continue with the troubleshooting.

>> Make sure you have your smartphone with you. Your Fitbit needs to have the smartphone close by to access the GPS signal.

>> Make sure your smartphone has Bluetooth enabled:

- *Android:* Tap Settings ⇨ Connections, and then tap the Bluetooth switch to On.

- *iOS:* Tap Settings ⇨ Bluetooth, and then tap the Bluetooth switch to on (green).

- *Windows 10:* Tap Start ⇨ Settings ⇨ Devices, make sure the Bluetooth and Other Devices tab is displayed, and then tap the Bluetooth switch to On.

>> Using the appropriate method in the preceding bullet, turn off your smartphone's Bluetooth setting, and then turn it back on again.

>> Make sure the exercise you've selected in the Exercise app has GPS turned on:

- *Charge 3:* Swipe up on the exercise screen to open the settings, and then tap the Use Phone GPS setting to On.

- *Versa:* In the exercise screen, tap the Settings icon (gear), and then tap the GPS setting to On.

>> Make sure Fitbit has permission to access your smartphone's GPS signal:

- *Android:* Tap Settings ⇨ Apps ⇨ Fitbit, tap Permissions, and then tap the Location switch to On.

- *iOS:* Tap Settings ⇨ Privacy ⇨ Location Services. Make sure the Location Services switch is on (green). Tap Fitbit and then tap While Using the App.

- *Windows 10:* Tap Start ⇨ Settings ⇨ Privacy ⇨ Location. Make sure the Allow Apps to Access Your Location switch is On. Then tap the Fitbit switch to On.

>> Restart your Fitbit, as I describe previously in the "Restarting your Fitbit" section.

>> Restart your smartphone.

Troubleshooting GPS with an Ionic

The Ionic watch has a built-in GPS chip, so you have full-time access to GPS through the Exercise app. Here are a few troubleshooting techniques to try if your Fitbit can't access GPS:

>> It sometimes takes a frustratingly long time for the Ionic to connect to GPS, so hang on for a minute or two before deciding to continue with the troubleshooting.

>> For best results when trying to establish a GPS connection, make sure you're outside and the watch is relatively still.

>> Make sure the exercise you've selected in the Exercise app has GPS turned on by swiping up and then tapping the GPS setting to On.

>> Restart your Fitbit, as I describe previously in the "Restarting your Fitbit" section.

Your Fitbit Device Was Submerged in Water

Your Fitbit fell in the water or was washed? First, ouch! Second, don't panic! Third, don't turn on your Fitbit! Fourth, do the following:

1. **Pour a cup or so of dry (that is, uncooked) rice into a sealable bag or jar.**

   Rice? Yep, rice is a natural drier-outer-of-things because it soaks up any surrounding moisture, including whatever moisture got into your Fitbit.

2. **Gently place your soggy Fitbit on top of the rice.**

3. **Close the bag or jar.**

4. **Leave the Fitbit with the rice for at least 24 hours.**

   If your Fitbit was submerged for a long time, you might want to leave it with the rice for 48 hours, just to make sure.

5. **Remove and then restart your Fitbit.**

   For details, see the "Restarting your Fitbit" section.

IN THIS CHAPTER

» **Protecting your Fitbit account with a super-duper password**

» **Looking for suspicious devices on your account**

» **Locking your Fitbit**

» **Locating a lost Fitbit**

» **Deleting your Fitbit data and activities**

Chapter **13**

Ten Ways to Improve Privacy and Security

You don't have to use your Fitbit for very long before you sense that there's something deeply *personal* about using one every day. Not only does your Fitbit account store sensitive details such as your birthday, height, and weight, but the more you use your tracker, the more personal data that gets stuffed into your account: activities, locations, sleep patterns, and much more. That's a big chunk of your personal life, so it pays to take whatever steps are required to keep that data safe and control who can see it and when.

In this chapter, you investigate ten ways to enhance the security and privacy of your Fitbit device, the Fitbit app, and your Fitbit account. Yep, it takes a bit of time to implement these measures, but that time is an excellent investment.

Protect Your Account with a Secure Password

Because everything you track with your device is tied to your Fitbit account, your tracking experience is only as secure as that account. Therefore, it's vital to ensure that you have your account locked down tight, and your first line of defense is a strong password. What do I mean by *strong*? For more info, check out the "Making up a strong password" sidebar. After you have a bulletproof password figured out, follow one of the procedures in this section to change your existing Fitbit password.

Changing your password by using the Fitbit app

Follow these steps to change your password by using the Fitbit app:

1. **Click Dashboard ⇨ Account.**

2. **Click Security and Login.**

3. **Click Change Password.**

   The Fitbit app displays the Change Password screen. Figure 13-1 shows the iOS version.

‹	Change Password	Change
Current Password	Old password	
New Password	New Password	
Confirm Password	Retype new password	
Your password must be at least 8 characters.		

FIGURE 13-1:
Use the Fitbit app's Change Password screen to update your Fitbit password.

4. **In the Current Password box, type your existing Fitbit account password.**

5. **In the New Password and Confirm Password boxes, type your new, strong password.**

   In the Android app, the second text box is named Confirm New Password.

6. **Click Change.**

   Fitbit updates your account with the new password.

Changing your password on Fitbit.com

Follow these steps to set a new password online by using the Fitbit.com website:

1. **Surf to www.fitbit.com and log in to your account.**

2. **Click the View Settings icon (gear), in the upper-right corner, and then click Settings.**

   Alternatively, you can surf directly to www.fitbit.com/settings/profile.

   The Personal Info tab is displayed by default. If you don't see that page, click Personal Info.

3. **Click Reset Password.**

   Fitbit sends an email with the subject Reset Your Fitbit Password to your address.

4. **Open the message and then click Reset Your Password.**

   Fitbit displays the Set Your Password page, shown in Figure 13-2.

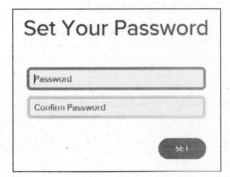

5. **In the Password and Confirm Password boxes, type your new, strong password.**

6. **Click Set.**

   Fitbit applies the new password to your account.

MAKING UP A STRONG PASSWORD

When it comes to securing your Fitbit account, it's not enough to just use any old password that pops into your head. To ensure the strongest security for your Fitbit data, make each password robust enough that it's impossible to guess and impervious to software programs designed to try different password combinations. Such a password is called a *strong password*. Ideally, you should build a password that provides maximum protection while still being easy to remember.

Lots of books will suggest ridiculously abstruse password schemes (I've written some of those books myself), but you really need to know only three things to create strong-like-a-bull passwords:

- **Use passwords that are at least 12 characters long.** Shorter passwords are susceptible to programs that just try every letter combination. You can combine the 26 letters of the alphabet into about 12 million five-letter word combinations, which is no big deal for a fast program. If you use 12-letter passwords — as many experts recommend — the number of combinations goes beyond mind-boggling: 90 quadrillion, or 90,000 trillion!

- **Mix up your character types.** Another secret to a strong password is to include characters from the following categories: lowercase letters, uppercase letters, punctuation marks, numbers, and symbols. If you include at least one character from three (or, even better, all five) of these categories, you're well on your way to a strong password.

- **Don't be obvious.** Because forgetting a password is inconvenient, many people use meaningful words or numbers so that their passwords will be easier to remember. Unfortunately, they often use obvious things such as their name, the name of a family member, pet, or colleague, their birth dates, or their Social Security number. Being this approach is just asking for trouble. Adding 123 or ! to the end of the password doesn't help much either because password-cracking programs try those.

Check Devices Logged In to Your Fitbit Account

Even with your Fitbit account locked down behind a strong password, a nefarious user might still gain access to the account. The most common way that someone can gain access is if you use the same login credentials on another website and that site is hacked and its users' login data stolen. That data is then usually sold or posted online, and before long some stranger logs in to your formerly secure Fitbit account.

If you want to check whether your Fitbit login credentials have been compromised, go to Have I Been Pwned? (*pwned* — it's pronounced "owned" — is hacker-speak for having been defeated or controlled by someone else) site at `https://haveibeenpwned.com/` and then enter your Fitbit login email address.

Other than voyeurism, which is bad enough, the only other reason someone might want access to your account is to mess with it by changing your settings, posting offensive messages to the community, or deleting your data.

You certainly don't want any unauthorized reprobate to access your account, so you should do two things:

>> Use a unique password for your Fitbit account.

>> Periodically check your account to see whether a device you don't recognize has logged in to the account.

The next two sections show you how to check which devices are logged in to your account by using the Fitbit app and the Fitbit.com website.

If you end up revoking access for a suspicious device, note that Fitbit only logs the device out of your account; it doesn't prevent the miscreant from logging in again. Therefore, as soon as you've revoked a device's access, run — I repeat, *run* — to the Change Password feature, as I described previously in the "Protect Your Account with a Secure Password" section. Your Fitbit account has been compromised, so the sooner you change your password, the better.

Checking logged in devices by using the Fitbit app

To use the Fitbit app to check the devices that are currently logged in, follow these steps:

1. **Click Dashboard ➪ Account.**

2. **Click Security and Login.**

3. **Click Manage Account Access.**

   Fitbit displays the Account Access screen, which lists all devices currently logged in to your Fitbit account.

4. **If you don't recognize a device, click the device to see more info.**

   Fitbit expands the device entry to display information such as the device model or web browser and the user's country.

5. **If the device looks suspicious, or if you're just not sure whether to trust it, click Revoke Access.**

   Fitbit asks you to confirm that you want to revoke access for the device.

6. **Click Confirm.**

   Fitbit revokes access to the device.

Checking logged in devices on Fitbit.com

To use Fitbit.com to check the devices that are currently logged in, follow these steps:

1. **Surf to www.fitbit.com and log in to your account.**

2. **Click View Settings ⇨ Settings.**

3. **Click the Manage Account Access tab.**

   You can also steer your web browser directly to www.fitbit.com/settings/data/access.

   You see the Account Access page, which lists all devices currently logged in to your Fitbit account.

4. **If you don't recognize a device, click the device to see more info.**

   Fitbit.com expands the device entry to display information such as the device model or web browser and the user's country. Figure 13-3 shows an example.

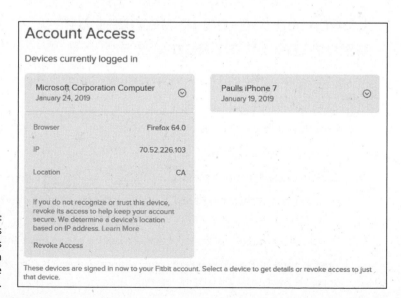

FIGURE 13-3:
On Fitbit.com's Account Access page, click a logged-in device to get more info.

5. **If the device looks suspicious, or if you're just not sure whether to trust it, click Revoke Access.**

   Fitbit.com asks you to confirm that you want to revoke access for the device.

6. **Click Confirm.**

   Fitbit.com revokes access to the device.

Control Which Data Can Be Seen By Friends and the Public

Your Fitbit tracker and your Fitbit account contain a ton of sensitive data, including personal data such as your birthday and gender, stats such as your steps taken and badges earned, and historical data such as graphs of your steps, calories, sleep, and weight. Fitbit also offers an engaging set of social features, as I describe in Chapter 4. Normally, combining sensitive data with social features is a privacy nightmare come true, but fortunately Fitbit comes with a decent set of tools that enable you to choose what you share and with whom.

For privacy purposes, Fitbit divides your world into three sharing categories:

>> **Private:** The data can be seen by only you (or anyone who can log in to your Fitbit account).

>> **Friends:** The data can be seen by only you and each person to whom you've connected as a Fitbit friend.

>> **Public:** The data can be seen by anyone, even people who don't have a Fitbit account.

Fitbit applies default privacy settings for data such as your birthday (Private), badges you've earned (Friends Only), and who you're friends with (Public). Use the steps in the next two sections to customize these and other privacy settings.

Customizing privacy settings by using the Fitbit app

To use the Fitbit app to customize your privacy settings, follow these steps:

1. **Click Dashboard ⇨ Account.**

2. **Click Privacy.**

   The Privacy screen appears. Figure 13-4 shows the iOS version.

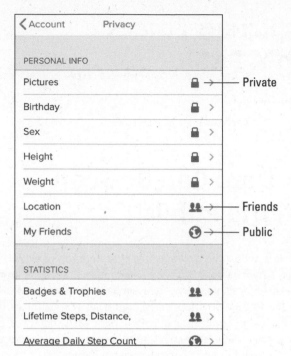

FIGURE 13-4:
Use the Privacy
screen to set
custom privacy
settings for your
Fitbit data.

3. **For each privacy setting, click the setting and then select Private, Friends, or Public.**

4. **(iOS only). After you select a different privacy option, you need to tap Save to put the change into effect.**

Customizing privacy settings on Fitbit.com

To use Fitbit.com to customize your privacy settings, follow these steps:

1. **Surf to www.fitbit.com and log in to your account.**

2. **Click View Settings ⇨ Settings.**

3. **Click Privacy.**

   You can also send your web browser directly to www.fitbit.com/settings/privacy.

4. **For each privacy setting, click the setting and then select Private, Friends, or Public.**

Beware of Suspicious Emails Supposedly from Fitbit

In recent years, Fitbit has seen an increase in fraudulent activity — mostly scammers who take over an account, request a replacement device from Fitbit, and then sell that device for a quick profit. How can someone take over your Fitbit account? The two main ways follow:

>> If your Fitbit account uses the same login credentials as one or more of your other online accounts, and at least one of those other accounts suffered a data breach that exposed your credentials, a scammer could use the stolen credentials to access your Fitbit account. If your credentials have been compromised (as I mention earlier, you can go to https://haveibeenpwned.com to check this), immediately change your Fitbit password. (See "Protect Your Account with a Secure Password," previously in this chapter.).

>> A scammer sends out a fraudulent email message that appears to come from Fitbit but is really a convincing fake created by the scammer. The most common of these is a "Password Reset Request" email, which provides a link where you can reset your Fitbit password. The link takes you to a page monitored by the scammer and used to harvest your Fitbit account password. Here are some tips to keep yourself safe from this type of phishing exploit:

   • If an email asks you to reset your password but you didn't initiate that request, it's almost certainly a scam. I say *almost* because Fitbit will send out a legit password reset request if it determines that your account has been hacked.

   • Before clicking any link related to your Fitbit account, hover your mouse pointer over the link to examine the link address. (On a mobile device, tap and hold down on the link to see a pop-up with the link address). If the address doesn't start with https://*subdomain*.fitbit.com (where *subdomain* is something like www, help, or dev), delete the email immediately.

   • If you end up on a website that asks for your Fitbit account credentials, check the address bar before entering any data. Again, if the address doesn't start with https://*subdomain*.fitbit.com, get out of there as fast as your browser's legs will take you.

Block or Remove a Fitbit User

If you've tried out any of the Fitbit social features that I went on and on about in Chapter 4, you already know that the Fitbit community is a welcoming, supportive bunch. You might already have made quite a few new friends. However, within any group of people, no matter how amiable and helpful that group might be overall, there will always be one or two bad seeds. It might be Boring Bill who goes on and on about nothing or Insufferable Sue who boasts about even the most minor accomplishment. Or it might be something more serious, such as someone who sends you vaguely (or even overtly) creepy or menacing messages.

Depending on the seriousness of the offence, you can handle the user in one two ways:

>> **Block the friend:** This temporarily removes the person as your friend and prevents the user from sending you messages and friend requests. Blocking a friend is the route to take if you just want to take a break from someone for a while. You can reinstate the user without having to send a new friend request.

>> **Remove the friend:** This permanently removes the person as your friend, which means he or she can no longer send you messages. Removing a friend is the route to take if you want someone out of your Fitbit life completely. The only way to reinstate the user is to send a new friend request.

Blocking or removing a friend by using the Fitbit app

To block or remove someone, follow these steps:

1. **Tap Community.**

2. **Tap the Friends tab.**

   Fitbit displays a list of your friends.

3. **Tap the friend you want to block or remove.**

   Fitbit displays the user's profile.

4. **Tap the More icon (three dots), in the upper-right corner (Android or iOS) or the lower-right corner (Windows 10).**

5. **Tap a command:**

- *Block Friend:* Tap this command to block the friend temporarily. When Fitbit asks you to confirm, tap OK.

- *Remove Friend:* Tap this command to remove the friend completely. Note that Fitbit doesn't ask for confirmation, so be sure this is what you want to do before tapping the Remove Friend command.

REMEMBER

To unblock a friend by using the Fitbit app (any version), click Dashboard ⇨ Account ⇨ Blocked Users, Then click the user you want to unblock, and click Add Friend. When Fitbit asks you to confirm, click OK.

Removing a friend on Fitbit.com

To use Fitbit.com to remove a Fitbit user (there's no online option to block someone), follow these steps:

1. **Surf to www.fitbit.com and log in to your account to display the Dashboard.**

2. **Hover your mouse pointer over the Friends tile and then click See More.**

    You can also send your web browser directly to www.fitbit.com/friends.

3. **Click the friend you want to remove.**

4. **Hover your mouse pointer over the teal Friends button.**

    The button turns red and the check mark turns into an X.

5. **Click Friends.**

    Fitbit asks you to confirm that you want to remove the friend.

6. **Click OK.**

    Fitbit removes the friend from your profile.

Lock Your Fitbit Device

If you have an Ionic watch, or a Charge 3 wristband or Versa watch with an NFC (near-field communication) chip, you have access to Fitbit Pay, which enables you to make contactless payments with your device. Fitbit Pay is convenient, but here's the thing: If you can make contactless payments with your Fitbit, so can someone else who steals or finds your lost device.

Similarly, a stolen or lost Fitbit contains lots of personal data about you that you probably don't want someone else to examine.

Whatever the reason, you can prevent unauthorized use or viewing of your Fitbit by locking the device with a four-digit PIN code. When your Fitbit is locked, the only way to access it is by entering the PIN code at least once each day (usually when you place the device on your wrist).

If you're already using Fitbit Pay, Fitbit would have prompted you to enter a PIN code when you configured Fitbit Pay for the first time. If not, you can follow these steps to lock your Fitbit with a PIN code:

1. **In the Fitbit app, click Dashboard ⇨ Account.**

2. **Click Device Lock.**

   If you don't see the Device Lock setting, your Fitbit doesn't support this feature.

3. **Click Set PIN Code.**

4. **Enter the four-digit code you want to use.**

5. **Enter the four-digit code a second time.**

   Fitbit enables the PIN and applies Device Lock to your Fitbit.

Here are the techniques to use if you need to modify Device Lock in some way:

>> **Entering a new pin:** In the Fitbit app, click Dashboard ⇨ Account ⇨ Device Lock and then click Change PIN.

>> **Disabling Device Lock:** In the Fitbit app, click Dashboard ⇨ Account ⇨ Device Lock and then click Disabled.

Locate a Lost Fitbit Device

Losing your Fitbit is a drag not only because you paid good money for the device but also because of the worry that someone else will find it. Unfortunately, Fitbit doesn't offer a special feature for locating a lost tracker, but you can try a few things:

>> In the Fitbit app, open the Dashboard, click Account, and then click your Fitbit. Check out the Synced value, shown in Figure 13-5. If it says *Synced today* and the sync time is recent, your Fitbit is within range of the device on which you're running the Fitbit app. Start looking!

FIGURE 13-5:
If you see a
recent sync time,
it means your
Fitbit is nearby.

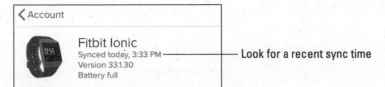

‹ Account

Fitbit Ionic
Synced today, 3:33 PM ——————— Look for a recent sync time
Version 33.1.30
Battery full

>> If you have a general idea where you lost your Fitbit, take the device on which you're running the Fitbit app to that area and then try syncing the Fitbit. If the sync works, it means your Fitbit is within about 33 feet of your location. It has to be around there somewhere!

>> Install and run a Bluetooth locator app, which is designed to sniff out nearby Bluetooth devices. For Android, check out Find My Device or Bluetooth Finder; for iOS, try Find Bluetooth or Find My Fitbit.

Delete Fitbit Data and Activities

I've talked about deleting Fitbit data throughout this book, mostly in the context of removing unneeded or erroneous entries. However, deleting data also has a privacy side, particularly when other people have access to your account. Because I've covered data deletion elsewhere in the book, I just give you a quick summary of the techniques here.

Deleting data using the Fitbit app

To use the Fitbit app to delete log entries, follow these steps:

1. **Display the Dashboard.**

2. **To delete a food entry:**

   a. *Click the Food Plan tile.*

   b. *Click the entry you want to remove.*

   c. *(Android or iOS) Tap the More icon (three dots), in the upper-right corner.*

   d. *Click Delete Log.*

3. **To delete an activity or exercise session:**

   a. *Click the Weekly Exercise tile.*

   b. *Click the entry you want to remove.*

   c. *(Android or iOS) Tap the More icon (three dots).*

   d. *Click Delete Exercise.*

4. **To delete a weigh-in:**

   a. *Click the Weight tile.*

   b. *Click the entry you want to remove.*

   c. *(Android or iOS) Tap the More icon (three dots).*

   d. *Click Delete Log.*

5. **To delete a sleep:**

   a. *Click the Sleep tile.*

   b. *Click the entry you want to remove.*

   c. *(Android or iOS) Tap the More icon (three dots).*

   d. *Click Delete Sleep Log.*

Deleting data on Fitbit.com

To use Fitbit.com to delete activities, weigh-ins, and other log data, follow these steps:

1. **Head over to www.fitbit.com and log in to your account.**

2. **In the main navigation header, click Log In.**

3. **To delete a food entry:**

   a. *Click the Food tab.*

   b. *Move the mouse pointer over the entry you want to remove.*

   c. *Click the Delete icon (X) that appears to the left of the entry.*

4. **To delete an activity or exercise session:**

   a. *Click the Activities tab.*

   b. *Move the mouse pointer over the entry you want to remove.*

   c. *Click the Delete icon (trash can) that appears to the right of the entry.*

   d. *Click Delete when Fitbit asks you to confirm.*

5. **To delete a weigh-in:**

   a. *Click the Weight tab.*

   b. *Click the Delete icon (trash can) that appears in the entry you want to remove.*

   c. *Click Confirm when Fitbit asks if you're sure.*

6. **To delete a sleep:**

   a. *Click the Sleep tab.*

   a. *Click the entry you want to remove.*

   a. *Click Delete.*

   b. *Click Delete Entry when Fitbit asks for confirmation.*

Erase All Your Fitbit Data

If you're selling or giving away your Fitbit, make sure the device is wiped clean of all your custom settings and personal info. You can erase your device data by resetting your Fitbit, which I describe in Chapter 12.

You also want to ensure that the device is no longer connected to your Fitbit account, and that means removing the device from your account. To learn how to remove a device, see Chapter 3.

Delete Your Fitbit Account

If you ever decide that Fitbit is no longer your thing, don't just throw your tracker in the nearest junk drawer. Make sure you also delete your Fitbit account, because that account probably has a ton of personal data about you that you don't want hanging around.

Note that Fitbit doesn't delete all that data right away. The Fitbit folks, ever optimistic, give you a bit of time to change your mind without losing your data. Here's the timeline Fitbit follows after you delete your account:

» **Up to 7 days:** Fitbit doesn't do anything with your account, just in case you have a change of heart. If you log in any time during the first 7 days, Fitbit asks if you want to cancel the deletion request and, if you say yes, will restore your account, no hard feelings.

>> **Between 8 and 30 days:** Fitbit freezes your account and begins deleting your data. Most of your data is deleted by the time the first 30 days are up.

>> **More than 30 days:** Fitbit continues deleting your data from backups and other sources. It might take as long as 90 days before all your data is electronic dust in the wind.

You can use either of the following techniques to request that your account be deleted:

>> **Fitbit app:** Click Dashboard ⇨ Account, and then click Manage Data. Click Delete Account, and then click Delete Account (Android) or Delete My Account & Data (iOS or Windows 10).

>> **Fitbit.com:** Log in and click View Settings ⇨ Settings. Click Delete Account, enter your account password, and then click Send Confirmation Email.

Chapter 14

Ten Ways to Connect to Third Parties

When you monitor your personal stats throughout the day by using your Fitbit device, the Fitbit app, and the Fitbit.com online Dashboard, it's easy to fall into a Fitbit-only mindset. Being stuck in Fitbit-land isn't a terrible thing because your Fitbit and its associated software can tell you a ton about your fitness and health and how it's progressing. That said, it's a big world out there and Fitbit isn't the only fitness and health game in town. There are other apps such as Strava and Weight Watchers; there are other devices such as Alexa and Cortana; and there are other types of content, such as music and podcasts.

Fortunately, because Fitbit is by far the most popular activity tracking company, many third parties have been eager to set up ways to connect their products to the Fitbit ecosystem. In this chapter, you explore the myriad ways that you can connect your Fitbit to these third-party apps, devices, and content.

Share Fitbit Data on Strava

As I show in Chapter 4, it's easy to connect with friends and groups to share your latest and greatest achievements. But if you're a dedicated exerciser or athlete, chances are you already have an account on Strava, which means it probably makes more sense to share data between your Fitbit account and your Strava account.

After you connect Fitbit and Strava, two things happen:

>> All GPS-related activities that you track with your Fitbit are synced to your Strava account.

>> All the activities that you track via Strava are added to your daily and weekly Fitbit stats.

Note that none of the preceding includes activities prior to making the connection between your two accounts. If you want to get your historical Fitbit data into Strava, you need to export the data, as I describe later in the "Export Your Fitbit Data" section.

REMEMBER

If you have a Fitbit watch, open the Strava app to see your ten most recent runs or rides.

Connecting Fitbit and Strava by using the Strava app

To connect your Fitbit and Strava accounts by using the Strava app, follow these steps:

1. Get started in the Strava app:

- *Android:* Tap Menu ⇨ Settings ⇨ Link Other Services. Then tap Connect a Device to Strava.

- *iOS:* Tap More ⇨ Settings ⇨ Applications, Services, and Devices. Then tap Connect a New Device to Strava.

2. Tap Fitbit.

3. Tap Connect Fitbit.

Strava prompts you to log in to your Fitbit account.

4. Type your Fitbit email address and password, and then tap Log In.

Strava prompts you to log in to your Strava account.

5. Type your Strava email address and password, and then tap Log In.

6. Tap Authorize.

Fitbit asks you to choose which data you want to allow Strava to access, as shown in Figure 14-1.

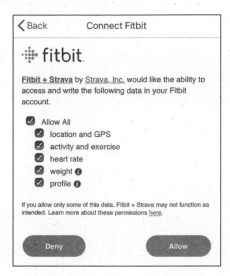

7. **Tap the Allow All check box.**

Note that you don't have to share everything with Strava. For example, there's probably not much point sharing your weight or your Fitbit profile with Strava.

8. **Tap to deselect the check box beside each item you don't want to share.**

9. **Tap the Allow button.**

Strava displays an overview of the sharing process.

10. **Tap OK, Got It.**

11. **Tap Done.**

Fitbit and Strava share any GPS-based activities that you track with one or the other.

Connecting Fitbit and Strava on the web

To connect Fitbit and Strava online by using a web browser, follow these steps:

1. **Surf to** https://strava.fitbit.com.

2. **Click Connect.**

Strava prompts you to authorize Fitbit to connect to Strava.

3. **Click Authorize.**

Fitbit prompts you to log in to your Fitbit account.

4. **Type your Fitbit email address and password, and then tap Log In.**

   Fitbit asks you to choose which data you want to allow Strava to access.

5. **Click the Allow All check box (or select the check box beside only those items you want to share), and then tap the Allow button.**

   Strava displays an overview of the sharing process.

6. **Click OK, Got It.**

   Fitbit and Strava share any GPS-based activities that you track with one or the other.

Share Fitbit Data on Weight Watchers

If you're a member of Weight Watchers, wouldn't it be great if you could convert your Fitbit activities into Weight Watchers activity points, or FitPoints in Weight Watchers lingo? Why, yes, it would — and you can. Just connect your Fitbit account with your Weight Watchers account and your Fitbit activities will be automatically synced to your Weight Watchers profile. Sweet!

Connecting Fitbit and Weight Watchers by using the Weight Watchers app

To connect your Fitbit and Weight Watchers accounts by using the Weight Watchers app, follow these steps:

1. **Get started in the Weight Watchers app:**

   - *Android:* Tap Profile ⇨ Settings. Then tap Activity Settings ⇨ Activity Sync.

   - *iOS:* Tap Profile ⇨ Settings. Then tap Activity Settings ⇨ Device.

2. **To connect a Fitbit activity tracker, tap Device.**

   To connect a Fitbit Aria 2 smart scale, tap Wireless Scale.

3. **Tap Fitbit.**

   Weight Watchers prompts you to log in to your Fitbit account.

4. **Type your Fitbit email address and password, and then tap Log In.**

   Fitbit asks you to choose which data you want to allow Weight Watchers to access (refer to Figure 14-1).

5. **Tap the Allow All check box.**

   Note that you don't have to share everything with Weight Watchers. For example, there's probably not much point sharing your sleep, your friends, or your Fitbit profile with Weight Watchers.

6. **Tap to deselect the check box beside each item you don't want to share.**

7. **Tap the Allow button.**

   Fitbit shares the data you selected with your Weight Watchers account.

Connecting Fitbit and Weight Watchers on the web

To connect your Fitbit and Weight Watchers accounts online by using a web browser, follow these steps:

1. **Surf to** `https://weightwatchers.com/`.

   If you're in Canada, go to `https://weightwatchers.ca`; for the UK, go to `https://weightwatchers.co.uk`.

2. **Log in to your account.**

3. **Click Account ⇨ Settings.**

4. **Click Device.**

   If you've previously connected a device with your Weight Watchers account, you need to remove it because Weight Watchers allows only one connected device at a time. To remove the device, click the Device logo or click Disconnect.

   Fitbit prompts you to log in to your Fitbit account.

5. **Type your Fitbit email address and password, and then tap Log In.**

   Fitbit asks you to choose which data you want to allow Weight Watchers to access.

6. **Click the Allow All check box (or select the check box beside only those items you want to share), and then tap Allow.**

   Fitbit shares the data you selected in Step 6 with your Weight Watchers account.

To get your Fitbit data synced to your Weight Watchers profile right away (and any time you feel like it), click Menu ⇨ My Day. Next, click the Activity tab, and then click the Sync with Your Fitbit App link, which appears at the bottom of the Activity tab (see Figure 14-2).

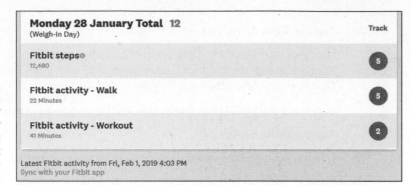

FIGURE 14-2:
On the My Day page's Activity tab, click Sync with Your Fitbit App to get the latest Fitbit data.

Share Fitbit Data with MyFitnessPal

MyFitnessPal is a calorie-counting app that enables you to track food (calories in) and exercises (calories out) to achieve a goal weight. It's one of the most popular health and fitness apps, and you can connect it to your Fitbit for easier tracking.

Connecting Fitbit and MyFitnessPal by using the MyFitnessPal app

Follow these steps to connect your Fitbit and MyFitnessPal accounts by using the MyFitnessPal app:

1. **Get started in the MyFitnessPal app:**

   - *Android:* Tap Menu ⇨ Apps and Devices.

   - *iOS:* Tap More ⇨ Apps and Devices.

2. **Tap Fitbit Tracker.**

3. **Tap Connect.**

   MyFitnessPal prompts you to log in to your MyFitnessPal account.

4. **Type your MyFitnessPal email address and password, and then tap Log In.**

   MyFitnessPal prompts you to log in to your Fitbit account.

5. **Type your Fitbit email address and password, and then tap Log In.**

   Fitbit asks you to choose which data you want to allow MyFitnessPal to access (refer to Figure 14-1).

6. **Tap Allow All.**

Unfortunately, MyFitnessPal insists that you share all your Fitbit data. If you try to share only some data, the connection with fail. Boo, MyFitnessPal!

7. **Tap Allow.**

Fitbit will now share your data with your MyFitnessPal account.

Connecting Fitbit and MyFitnessPal on the web

To connect your Fitbit and MyFitnessPal accounts online using a web browser, follow these steps:

1. **Surf to** https://myfitnesspal.com/ **and then log in to your account.**

2. **Click Apps.**

3. **Click Fitbit Tracker.**

4. **Click Connect.**

5. **If prompted, type your Fitbit email address and password, and then tap Log In.**

Fitbit asks you to choose which data you want to allow MyFitnessPal to access (refer to Figure 14-1).

6. **Click the Allow All check box and then click the Allow button.**

Fitbit now shares your data with your MyFitnessPal account.

Share Fitbit Data with Other Apps

In the previous three sections I talk about the specific steps to take to connect your Fitbit device and account with three apps: Strava, Weight Watchers, and MyFitnessPal. However, Fitbit trackers are so popular that just about every fitness, health, diet, and weight loss app offers a way to connect to a Fitbit device. To give you an idea, Table 14-1 offers a list of the apps that have official ties to Fitbit (current as of this writing).

TABLE 14-1 Apps That Work with Fitbit

App	Category	Website
Dick's Sporting Goods	Health	www.dickssportinggoods.com
Endomondo	Fitness	www.endomondo.com
Fitabase	Health	https://www.fitabase.com
Fitline	Fitness	http://geekutils.com
FitTap	Health	www.fittap.it
Fitwatchr	Diet and weight loss	www.fitwatchr.com
Habit	Diet and weight loss	https://habit.com
LFconnect	Fitness	https://lifefitness.com
Lose It!	Diet and weight loss	www.loseit.com
MapMyRun	Fitness	www.mapmyrun.com
MINDBODY	Health	www.mindbodyonline.com
MyNetDiary	Diet and weight loss	www.mynetdiary.com
Nudge Health Tracking	Fitness	https://nudgecoach.com/nudgeapp/
Peloton	Fitness	www.onepeloton.ca
RunKeeper	Fitness	https://runkeeper.com
Running for Weight Loss	Diet and weight loss	Search your device app store
SparkPeople	Fitness	www.sparkpeople.com
Stridekick	Fitness	https://stridekick.com
Tactio Health	Health	www.tactiohealth.com
Thermos Hydration Bottle with Smart Lid	Diet and weight loss	www.thermos.com/smartlid
Trainerize	Fitness	www.trainerize.com
TrainingPeaks	Fitness	www.trainingpeaks.com

App	Category	Website
Trendweight	Diet and weight loss	https://trendweight.com
VirZOOM	Fitness	www.virzoom.com
Walgreens Balance Rewards	Health	www.walgreens.com/balancerewards/balance-rewards.jsp
Walkadoo	Fitness	https://walkadoo.meyouhealth.com
Waterlogged	Diet and weight loss	www.waterlogged.com
Wokamon	Fitness	www.wokamon.com

Yep: that's a lot of apps! Unfortunately, I can't offer a one-size-fits-all method that enables you to connect any one of these apps to your Fitbit device and account. However, I can do the next best thing and offer a general procedure to try for any app:

>> **Using the third-party's app:** Open the app's Settings or main menu, and then look for a command named something like Apps, Devices, or Connect. Click Fitbit, log in to your Fitbit account if asked, and then choose which data you want to share with the app by using the screen shown previously in Figure 14-1.

>> **Using the third party's website:** Log in to your app account. Open the site's main menu, and then look for a command named something like Apps, Devices, or Connect. Click Fitbit, log in to your Fitbit account if asked, and then choose which data you want to share with the app by using the screen shown previously in Figure 14-1.

Export Your Fitbit Data

Fitbits are so popular that almost all major fitness- and health-related apps and services have an option to connect to your Fitbit account. However, you might be using an app or service that doesn't offer such a connection. Are you out of luck? Perhaps not. Fitbit offers a couple of ways to export your data to a file. If your app or service has a method for importing files, you might be able to import your Fitbit data.

Fitbit offers two types of file exports:

>> **Single activity TCX file:** This Training Center XML (TCX) file includes the GPS data for a run or other activity, as well as data related to the activity such as average heart rate and calories burned.

>> **All activities ZIP file:** This archive (ZIP) file contains all your Fitbit data. Most of the data comes as either a JavaScript object notation (JSON) file or a comma separated values (CSV) file.

In practice, you'll almost always want a TCX file to import into a service. However, I also include the instructions for exporting all your data, just in case you want a record of what Fitbit has stored for you.

Export an activity as a TCX file

To export a GPS-tracked activity as a TCX file, follow these steps:

1. **Surf to www.fitbit.com and log in to open your Dashboard.**

2. **In the navigation bar, click Log.**

3. **Click Activities.**

4. **Locate the GPS-tracked activity you want to export, and then click the activity's View Details button.**

5. **Click the More icon, labeled in Figure 14-3, and then click Export as TCX file.**

   Fitbit gathers the activity's data into a TCX file and then downloads that file to your PC.

TIP

As an alternative to Steps 1 through 3, you can head directly to your Activities log by going to www.fitbit.com/activities.

Export all your Fitbit activities

To export all your Fitbit data, follow these steps:

1. **Point your web browser to www.fitbit.com and log in to open your Dashboard.**

2. **Click View Settings ⇨ Settings.**

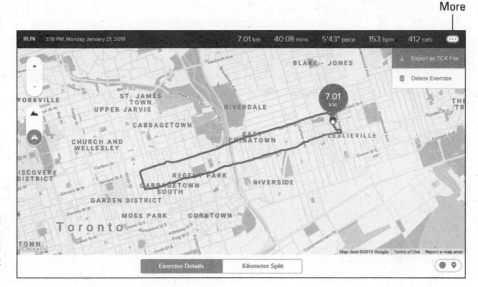

FIGURE 14-3:
Open the activity,
click More, and
then click Export
as TCX File.

3. **Click Data Export.**

   Fitbit opens the Export My Fitbit Data page.

   As an alternative to Steps 1 through 3, you can head directly to this page by going to www.fitbit.com/settings/data/export.

   TIP

4. **Click Request My Data.**

   Fitbit sends an email to your Fitbit address asking you to confirm your data request.

5. **In the Fitbit email, click Confirm Export Request.**

   Fitbit begins the process of exporting your data. In the Export My Fitbit Data page, you see a Current Export item with a percentage that tells you how far along things have progressed (see Figure 14-4). Click the Refresh icon to see the latest percentage.

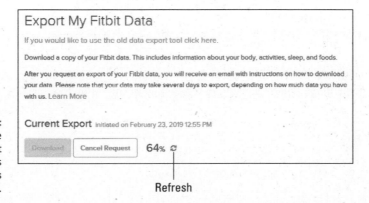

FIGURE 14-4:
The percentage
in the Current
Export item tells
you the progress
of your export.

Refresh

6. **When the export preparation is complete (that is, when the percentage in the Current Export item reaches 100), click the Download button.**

   Your web browser downloads the file, which is usually named MyFitBitData.zip.

Connect Fitbit to Alexa

If you have an Alexa-enabled device at home — such as an Amazon Echo or a third-party speaker that includes Alexa — you can ask Alexa for your current Fitbit stats, including steps taken, flights climbed, and your resting heart rate. To make Alexa Fitbit-aware, you must first enable the Fitbit skill on your Alexa device.

To enable the Fitbit skill with your voice, use either of the following commands:

"Alexa, enable Fitbit."

"Alexa, open Fitbit."

REMEMBER

If Alexa tells you it can't find the Fitbit skill, it likely means the skill is not available in your country. Fitbit adds new countries every so often, so keep trying to enable the skill once a month or so.

You can also enable the Fitbit skill using the Alexa app, as shown in the following steps:

1. **In the Alexa app, choose Menu ⇨ Skills & Games.**
2. **Click the Search icon (magnifying glass), and then type** fitbit **in the Search screen.**
3. **Tap the Fitbit skill to open its information page.**
4. **Tap Enable.**

   Alexa enables the skill.

With the Fitbit skill enabled, you invoke the skill by saying "Alexa, ask Fitbit *something*", where *something* can be any of the following:

>> How many steps I've taken today

>> How many flights I've climbed today

>> How many active minutes I have today

- >> How many calories I've burned today

- >> How far I've walked today

- >> How I'm doing today

- >> How I slept last night

- >> If I've exercised today

- >> How much water I've had today

- >> What my resting heart rate is

- >> How much I weigh

- >> About my battery

Connect Fitbit to Window 10's Cortana

If you a Cortana-enabled Windows 10 device, you can ask Cortana to tell you your current Fitbit stats, including steps taken, flights climbed, and your resting heart rate. To get Cortana connected to Fitbit, you must first enable the Fitbit skill on your Windows 10 device.

To enable the Fitbit skill, issue the following command:

"Cortana, ask Fitbit."

With the Fitbit skill enabled, you invoke the skill by saying "Cortana, ask Fitbit *something*", where *something* can be any of the following:

- >> How many steps I've taken today

- >> How many flights I've climbed today

- >> How many active minutes I have today

- >> How many calories I've burned today

- >> How far I've walked today

- >> How I'm doing today

- >> How I slept last night

>> If I've exercised today

>> How much water I've had today

>> What my resting heart rate is

>> How much I weigh

>> About my battery

Get the Weather on Your Fitbit

If your Fitbit supports apps, one of those apps is called Weather, which can put the current conditions right there on your wrist. Nice. First, though, you need to follow these steps to configure your weather settings:

1. **Click Dashboard ➪ Account.**

2. **Click your Fitbit device.**

3. **Click Apps.**

    If you don't see the Apps icon, your Fitbit doesn't support running apps.

4. **Click the Settings icon (gear) next to the Weather app.**

    Fitbit displays the Weather app's Settings screen, shown in Figure 14-5.

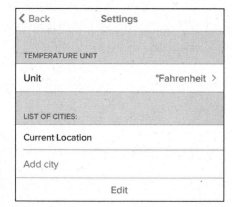

FIGURE 14-5:
The Settings screen for the Weather app.

5. **To change the temperature unit, click Unit and then click either Fahrenheit or Celsius.**

6. **To add a city to the Weather app:**

   a. *Click Add City.*

   b. *Start typing the name of the city.*

   c. *Click the full name of the city when it appears in Fitbit's list of cities that match what you've typed so far.*

7. **Click the Back icon (<) until you return to the Account screen.**

   Fitbit syncs the new settings to the Weather app.

REMEMBER

If you add multiple cities to the Weather app, you can switch between cities in the app by swiping left or right.

Listen to Audio on Your Fitbit Watch

If you have an Ionic or Versa Fitbit watch, you can upload music and podcast playlists to your watch. Then, after you've connected a pair of Bluetooth headphones or speakers to the watch (see "Pair Bluetooth Headphones or Speakers," later in this chapter), you can use your Fitbit to control the playback of your tunes or podcasts.

Before getting started, make sure you've installed Fitbit on the computer that contains the music and podcast playlists you want to transfer to your watch:

>> **Windows 10:** You can use the Windows 10 version of the Fitbit app.

>> **Mac (or an older version of Windows 10 that can't run the Fitbit app):** You need to install Fitbit Connect, as I describe in Chapter 3.

Connecting your watch to Wi-Fi

The only way to upload audio playlists from your computer to your watch is through Wi-Fi, so your first chore is to connect your watch to the same Wi-Fi network that your PC or Mac is connected to. Follow these steps in the Fitbit app:

1. **Click Dashboard ⇨ Account.**

2. **Click your Fitbit watch.**

3. **Click the Media tile.**

4. **Click Manage Wi-Fi Networks.**

5. **(iOS only) Click Next.**

   The Wi-Fi Setup screen appears with a list of nearby networks.

6. **Click the Wi-Fi network you want to use.**

7. **Type the network password, and then click Connect.**

   Fitbit connects your watch to the Wi-Fi network.

Uploading playlists to your watch

With your computer and your Fitbit watch eyeballing each other across your Wi-Fi network, as I describe in the preceding section, you're ready to transfer a playlist or three to your watch. How you proceed depends on whether you're using Windows 10 or a Mac.

REMEMBER

You can transfer only playlists, not individual music tracks or podcast episodes. You can create on-the-fly playlists by using the Fitbit app or Fitbit Connect. However, you get more control if you create the playlists you want on your watch in advance by using Groove Music (Windows 10) or iTunes (Mac).

Uploading playlists from your Windows 10 PC

To transfer audio from your Windows 10 computer to your Fitbit watch, you use the Fitbit app. Follow these steps:

1. **In the main navigation bar at the top of the Fitbit app, click the Media icon (musical note).**

2. **Click Personal Music.**

   Fitbit sets up a connection with your watch, and then displays a list of your Groove Music playlists.

3. **Wake your Fitbit watch.**

4. **Swipe left until you see the Music app, and tap Music to open the screen shown in Figure 14-6.**

5. **Tap Transfer Music.**

   Later, after you've added one or more playlists, you'll need to scroll to the bottom of the Music app to see the Transfer Music button.

TIP

To create a new playlist by using the Fitbit app, click Create New Playlist, click the added playlist to open it, then drag music from Groove Music and drop it inside the playlist.

No Music Loaded

Use Fitbit desktop app to transfer music to Ionic.

Transfer Music

FIGURE 14-6:
To put your watch into Transfer Mode, tap Transfer Music.

6. **Select the check box for each playlist you want to transfer to your watch.**

WARNING

When you select a playlist, Fitbit immediately begins the process of uploading the audio! Therefore, don't select a playlist unless you're sure you want to upload it.

Depending on the number of music tracks and podcast episodes that you're uploading to your watch, it can take an hour or more to complete the transfer.

Keep your eye on the watch storage meter at the top of the Fitbit app window. When that meter is full, you can't add any more audio to your watch. The storage meter also doubles as a progress bar, displaying the progress of the transfer.

7. **When Fitbit completes the audio transfer, return to your Fitbit watch, open the Music app, and then tap End Now.**

You can now control audio playback on the Fitbit watch using the Music app.

Uploading playlists from your Mac

To get one or more iTunes playlists from your Mac to your Fitbit watch, you use the Fitbit Connect app. Here are the steps to follow:

1. **Launch Fitbit Connect on your Mac.**

2. **Click Manage My Music.**

Fitbit Connect prompts you to log in to your Fitbit account. Note that you don't see this prompt if you've previously logged in, so in that case you can skip to Step 4.

3. **Enter your Fitbit credentials, and then click Log In.**

Fitbit Connect tells you to initiate Transfer Mode on your watch.

4. **Wake your Fitbit watch.**

5. **Swipe left until you see the Music app, and then tap Music.**

6. **Tap Transfer Music (refer to Figure 14-6).**

   After you've added one or more playlists, you'll need to scroll to the bottom of the Music app to access the Transfer Music button.

   Fitbit Connect sets up a connection with your watch, and then displays a list of your iTunes playlists.

   TIP To create a new playlist from Fitbit Connect, click Create New Playlist, click the added playlist to open it, then drag music from iTunes and drop it inside the playlist.

7. **Select the check box for each playlist you want to transfer to your watch.**

   WARNING When you select a playlist, Fitbit Connect immediately starts uploading the audio! Therefore, don't select a playlist unless you're sure you want to upload it.

   Depending on the number of music tracks and podcast episodes you're uploading to your watch, the transfer can take an hour or more to complete.

   Keep your eye on the watch storage meter at the top of the Fitbit Connect window. When that meter is full, you can't add any more audio to your watch. The storage meter also doubles as a progress bar, displaying the progress of the transfer.

8. **When Fitbit Connect completes the music transfer, return to your Fitbit watch, open the Music app, and then tap End Now.**

   You can now control audio playback on your watch using the Music app.

Controlling audio on your watch

After you have your Fitbit watch loaded with your favorite audio (as described in the preceding section) and you've paired Bluetooth headphones or speakers with the watch (as described in the next section), you're ready to feel the noise.

To get started, wake your Fitbit watch, swipe left from the clock until you see the Music icon, and then tap Music.

To start some audio, use either of these techniques:

» Tap Shuffle All to play all your audio in random order.

» Tap a playlist to display its audio, then tap a track or episode.

To display the audio playback controls, you again have two choices:

>> Open the Music app, tap the current playlist, and then tap the current track.

>> Press and hold down the watch's Back button. If you don't see the audio playback controls, swipe right.

With the playback controls onscreen, you can pause and play the audio, skip to the next track (tap >>), return to the beginning of the current track (tap <<), skip to the previous track (tap << twice), increase the volume (tap +), or decrease the volume (tap –).

Pair Bluetooth Headphones or Speakers

Your Fitbit watch can play, pause, and stop audio, but if you want to *hear* what's being played (and I think you do), you need to connect your watch to headphones or speakers via Bluetooth. Here's how to do it:

1. **Put your Bluetooth headphones or speakers into pairing mode.**

See the manual that came with your headphones or speakers to learn how to put the device into pairing mode.

2. **Wake your Fitbit watch.**

3. **Swipe left from the clock until you see the Settings app, and then tap Settings.**

4. **Tap Bluetooth.**

5. **Tap + Audio Device.**

Your watch begins looking for nearby devices that are in pairing mode. When your watch locates your headphones or speakers, it displays the name of the device.

6. **Tap the device name.**

Your Fitbit watch pairs with the headphones and speakers.

Glossary

Okay, you're at a cocktail party and you want to humblebrag about your ridiculously high average daily step count, your impressively low resting heart rate, or some other Fitbit metric. Good luck with that! However, to make sure people know you walk the walk and not just talk the talk, you need to pepper your claims with a few choice words and phrases related to tracking. Here are a few to consider.

accelerometer: A special sensor inside each Fitbit that's designed to detect movement (especially acceleration) and convert that movement into data.

active minutes: At least ten minutes of an activity performed at *moderate intensity* or *vigorous intensity*.

activity tracker: A device (such as a Fitbit) that tracks your activities throughout the day, including steps taken, floors climbed, and distance covered.

adaptation: The process where, after exercise, your body doesn't just repair the damage; it rebuilds your heart and muscles so that they're stronger.

altimeter: A sensor inside most Fitbits that detects changes in elevation, which is how a Fitbit can detect *floors* climbed.

badge: An award bestowed by Fitbit when you achieve one of its defined milestones, such as 15,000 steps in a day (the Urban Boots badge) or 1,000 floors climbed since joining Fitbit (the Skydiver badge).

basal metabolic rate (BMR): The rate at which you burn calories to perform standard bodily functions such as your heartbeat, breathing, and brain activity.

body fat percentage: The amount of fat in your body divided by your total weight.

body mass index (BMI): A calculation that roughly shows your weight relative to your height.

calorie deficit: When the number of calories you consume is less than the number of calories you burn.

cardio fitness level: Where your *cardio fitness score* rates in relation to people of the same gender and age range.

cardio fitness score: Fitbit's estimate of your *VO2 max.*

cardio zone: A *heart rate zone* between 70 and 85 percent of your maximum heart rate.

challenge: A step-based competition to see who can take the most steps during a specified time.

cue: An update during a workout that gives you a kind of progress report, such as the total distance and pace every mile.

digital exhaust: The trackable or storable actions, choices, and preferences that you generate as you go about your life.

easy intensity: An energy expenditure rate of less than three *METs.*

exercise auto-recognition: A Fitbit feature that automatically recognizes when you're doing an exercise such as a walk, run, or bike ride.

exercise: A *moderate intensity* activity that lasts at least 15 minutes.

external motivation: Getting other people involved in firing yourself up to exercise, diet, and the like.

fat burn zone: A *heart rate zone* between 50 and 69 percent of your maximum heart rate.

floor: An increase in elevation of ten feet.

food plan: A weekly *calorie deficit* target designed to help you reach your goal weight.

guardian: A family account member who can add and remove other guardians, invite family members to join, and create accounts for children.

handedness: The hand that is your dominant hand.

heart rate monitor: A sensor that uses a *pulse oximeter* to measure heart rate.

heart rate reserve: The difference between your *maximum heart rate* and your *resting heart rate.*

heart rate variability (HRV): The beat-to-beat changes in your heart rate.

heart rate zone: A subrange of the *heart rate reserve* characterized by the level of exertion and how the body uses energy to power that activity.

hourly activity: Taking at least 250 steps each hour for a specified number of hours each day.

interval workout: An activity where you alternate periods of relatively hard effort with periods of relatively low effort (or even rest).

lean mass: A measurement of the non-fat parts of your body.

macroscope: The general term for any technology that enhances a person's ability to gather and analyze data.

maximum heart rate: The highest possible number of beats per minute you can achieve.

metabolic equivalent of task (MET): A measure used to compare the rate of energy expended during different types of activities. One MET is defined as the amount of energy you expend when you're at rest.

metabolic rate: The rate at which you burn calories for both standard bodily functions (*basal metabolic rate*) and activities such as walking and running.

metric: A standard that you use to measure something. In the Fitbit world, the number of steps you take or the number of floors you climb are examples of metrics.

moderate intensity: An energy expenditure rate of at least three *METs* but less than six METs.

optical heart rate monitor: See *heart rate monitor*.

peak zone: A *heart rate zone* over 85 percent of your maximum heart rate

pedometer: A device that automatically counts the number of steps you take.

photoplethysmography (PPG): A hard-to-pronounce method of measuring artery volume using light.

pulse oximeter: A device that both emits light and measures how much of the light is absorbed or reflected by the blood.

quantified self: The self-tracking movement. People in the movement are quantified selfers, or *QSers*

resting heart rate: Your lowest waking heart rate.

self-tracker: A person who uses technology to acquire, store, and analyze his or her own life data.

sleep cycle: A series of sleep stages, where each cycle can last up to 90 minutes.

sleep efficiency: The percentage of time in bed that you're asleep.

sleep pattern: The number of minutes or hours or both each night that you spend in each sleep state or sleep stage.

sleep quality: An overall measure of how well you sleep.

sleep stage: One of four types of sleep — light, deep, REM, or awake — characterized by a particular level of brain activity and heart rate.

sleep state: One of three sleep types — asleep, restless, or awake — monitored by Fitbits that lack a *heart rate monitor*.

vigorous intensity: An energy expenditure rate of at least six *METs*.

VO2 max: The maximum rate of oxygen consumption that occurs when a person performs exercise of increasing intensity.

Index

F

LFconnect app, 288
light sleep stage, 127
light-emitting diodes. *See* LEDs (light-emitting diodes)
locking Fitbit devices, 275–276
London badge, 122
Lose It! app, 288
lurkers, in groups, 91

M

Mac computers
    removing Fitbit devices from accounts on, 49
    uploading playlists to watches from, 297–298
    using Fitbit Connect on, 43–44
main activity goals, 99
MapMyRun app, 288
Marathon badge, 122
martial arts
    detecting heart rate during, 23
    trackers for, 38
maximal aerobic capacity. *See* VO2 max
maximal oxygen uptake. *See* VO2 max
maximum heart rate, determining, 156–157
measurement units, adjusting, 54–55
messaging
    with Fitbit app, 80
    replying, 81
    through website, 80–81
    viewing, 81
MET (metabolic equivalent of task)
    improving cardio fitness score with higher, 190
    overview, 110–112
metabolic rate, defined, 111
metrics
    adjusting measurement units, 54–55
    on Dashboard, 51
    fitness tracking, 17–25
        active minutes, 21–22
        calories burned, 23–24
        distance covered, 19–20
        floors climbed, 20–21
        heart rate, 22–23
        sleep time, 25
        steps taken, 17–18
    voice cues and, 196

miles, setting measurement units to, 54–55
MINDBODY app, 288
moderate intensity activity
    activities included as, 112
    defined, 111
motivation, 10–11
move periods, 200
music
    pairing bluetooth headphones or speakers, 299
    trackers accessing, 38
    uploading to watches, 296–298
        from Mac, 297–298
        from Windows 10 PC, 296–297
MyFitnessPal, 286–287
MyNetDiary app, 288

N

near-field communication (NFC) chips, 275
notifications
    customizing, 63–64
    disabling, 64
    firmware update available, 251
    low battery power, 257
    troubleshooting, 255–256
    turning off for sleeping, 132–133
Nudge Health Tracking app, 288

O

Olympian sandals badge, 122
100-pound weight loss badge, 122
online resources
    cheat sheet for this book, 3
    checking Fitbit login credentials, 269
    connecting Strava to Fitbit, 283–284
    Dick's Sporting Goods app, 288
    Endomondo app, 288
    Fitabase app, 288
    Fitbit wireless sync dongle, 48
    Fitline app, 288
    FitTap app, 288
    Fitwatchr app, 288
    Habit app, 288
    installing Fitbit Connect, 44

About the Author

Paul McFedries has been writing technical books since 1991 and has published more than 95 books that have sold over four million copies worldwide. Paul is a lifelong runner, hiker, and fitness nut with a fairly ridiculous collection of GPS watches, heart-rate monitors, fitness apps, and other health-related tracking gear. Paul is also the proprietor of Word Spy (www.wordspy.com), a website that has been tracking recently coined words and phrases since 1995. Paul invites everyone to drop by his personal website (www.mcfedries.com) or follow him on Twitter (@paulmcf and @wordspy).

Dedication

To Karen and Chase, who make life fun.

Author's Acknowledgments

Publishing a book is a 10,000-step process that, alas, doesn't count even a little to one's fitness and health goals. Unless you're talking about mental health — even though I've had lots of books published (closing in on 100!), I still get warm and decidedly fuzzy feelings when I hold a new book in my hands for the first time. That mood boost comes from a sense of accomplishment, of course, but those endorphins get released also because I know the book was a work of collaboration. Sure, I wrote the text and I took the screenshots, but those tasks represent only a small portion of what went into making the book. The rest of it is brought to you by the dedication and professionalism of Wiley's editorial and production teams, who toiled long and hard to turn my text and images into an actual book.

I offer my sincere gratitude to everyone at Wiley who made this book possible, but I'd like to extend a special "Thanks a million!" to the folks I worked with directly: associate publisher Katie Mohr and project editor Susan Pink. I'd also like to give a big shout-out to my agent, Carole Jelen, for helping to make this project possible.

Publisher's Acknowledgments

Associate Publisher: Katie Mohr

Project Editor: Susan Pink

Copy Editor: Susan Pink

Sr. Editorial Assistant: Cherie Case

Production Editor: Mohammed Zafar Ali

Cover Image: © Atanas Bezov/Shutterstock